First Admission

First

Admission

A Handbook to New Grad Nursing

Jaison Chahwala BSN, CCM.

[Foreword by Ebi of Nurselifern]

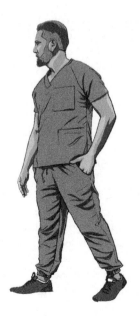

Send all love, hate, products, and anything else you can think of to:

First Admission
PO Box #1
Lemont, IL 60439

Media Requests/Speaking Engagements:
FirstAdmissionBook@Gmail.com

Follow:
Instagram: @FirstAdmission

We all strive to be *that* nurse.

You know, that one that likes to book vacations on company time, while their preceptee answers all of the call lights.

BEFORE YOU PUNCH IN

OKAY, HERE'S THE DEAL: THIS ISN'T JUST SOME run-of-the-mill nursing tell-all that will leave you feeling uneasy, angry, or proactive once you finish it. This also isn't your basic how-to manual that provides picture-perfect advice to ensure a lovely, everlasting career.

These are some of my experiences, which are going to be (or have been) some of your experiences too. No matter how unique each nurse's career may appear, you'll soon realize we can all relate closely to each other. As one of my favorite professors in nursing school once told me, "In nursing, concepts and principles are fixed on a continuum of changing nurses and landscapes. What you will go through is what he will go through, is what she will go through, and so on and so forth."

I wrote this handbook to serve as a guide and companion as you navigate your way through nursing school and into your career. My solutions may not work for everyone, and that's ok. What worked for me may help you decide what works for you. The chapter titles are self-explanatory, so feel free to skip around. Most importantly, enjoy the read.

CONTENTS

FOREWORD

BY EBI OF NURSELIFERN

FROM THE SECOND YOU'RE ACCEPTED **INTO NURSING SCHOOL** until the day you die, people will ask you the same two questions: What made you go into nursing, and why would you choose to do this to yourself? Well, maybe not that second question, but definitely the first is asked, and it's always bothered me.

I think part of the reason that first question bothers me is because I've never had the urge to do a deep dive into the personal life of someone I've just met and ask them why they became an accountant, or a chef, or a truck driver, or whatever. But somehow, every time I meet someone and mention I'm a nurse, it feels like they're expecting an origin story worthy of a comic book hero.

In this book Jaison chronicles his own origin story, as well as lessons learned along the way on his path to becoming a nurse. As I read through it, I couldn't help but reflect on my own path to becoming a nurse, and the themes that have run through my career from nursing school till today, ten years later.

Although not all my experiences line up with Jaison's, the book rings remarkably true and relatable to anyone who's ever worked a twelve-hour shift in a hospital and beyond. Jaison's blunt communication style and his cautious nature—bordering on paranoia—makes for the perfect guide book for students and new nurses.

So what if I chose to go into nursing for practical reasons? Perhaps for reasons that don't sound very heroic?

I was an average student in high school, and a bit of a class clown, but I always managed to absorb enough information to pass my tests while distracting my classmates. My grades were mostly Bs and Cs with a sprinkling of As. Basically, the best grades one could hope for without submitting much homework.

It wasn't until college that I decided to take my education more seriously, mostly because I had to pay for

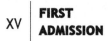

it on my own. Nothing brings you back to reality quicker than a student loan letter showing your ballooning account balance.

Heading into college, I already knew I'd major in nursing, simply because my mom had talked me into it. Growing up, she would ask me what I wanted to be when I got older. She would then promptly tell me how poor that profession would make me. Practicality was a big deal to her. I would not be surprised if my parents actively avoided exposing me to the arts, for fear that I would want to become a musician or something.

By the time I was a sophomore in college, the decision to become a nurse started to feel like my own. I learned more about nursing as a career, and a lot of it actually seemed like a great match for me. I loved science, I've always enjoyed working with people, and working three days a week (like most nurses) did not sound bad at all. Of course, I found out the hard way that three twelve-hour shifts a week is plenty. Despite this, I still loved the idea that I would have four days a week to myself to pursue other ventures. Seemed like a fair trade. None of this makes for a good origin story.

When people ask why I chose nursing, what they are really asking is, why did you gravitate to a profession that is known to be so physically and emotionally taxing? As much as the question bothers me, a part of me knows it makes sense.

Thinking of nursing as a calling is comforting for both nurse and patient.

If you're a patient who is having one of the worst days of your life, the thought of a literal godsend can be very comforting. If you're the nurse in this scenario, there's something comforting to you as well, in the idea that the universe or something greater put you in a position of being a safety net between life and death. Life and death bears a lot of responsibility for mere mortals, so naturally, nurses must be special.

This is why nurses tend to be a self-righteous bunch. It feels like an affront to push a narrative that suggests some random Joe Schmoe Nurse is trying to do both—make a living *and* be a great nurse— even though there is plenty of evidence that proves the two ideas are not antonymous of one another. One such piece of evidence to support this is the fact that a ton of *great* nurses *hate* their jobs. As enticing as being an angel or a superhero sounds, they don't get paid. Seems like I'm being facetious, but all these narratives are harmful to nurses and the nursing profession. Nothing makes this clearer than the transformation from the 7 p.m. applause at the start of the pandemic to the now far more popular "you signed up for this" comments. These comments are a clear and almost logical progression from hero worship to martyrdom. It is how every superhero movie ends. The hero sacrifices themselves, or at the very least puts themselves in harm's way, to save the general public. No nurse signed up for that.

I do genuinely believe that most people who go into nursing want to help people and aren't completely financially motivated. If it were about money, there are much less strenuous ways to make 50k a year (and yes, I am aware that salary varies wildly depending on where you live).

The idea I am trying to articulate is that when we lean too far into the "hero" aspects of our job and make it our whole identity, we risk being taken advantage of by our employers and being abused by the public. It's easy to abuse someone who is expected to sacrifice themselves for you, and it's easy to be stingy with wages when it's not a job but a calling.

It's always been a conscious decision on Nurselifern to push the conversation away from the caricatures of nursing and towards the realities. When we tell our stories, it humanizes us and it forces the public to see us as everyday people who need appropriate staffing and resources to do their job. Using our voices and platforms makes it difficult for us to be manipulated by our employers. Jaison's book is part of that storytelling and conversation that is moving nursing from its caricature to reality.

Whether you're in your first semester of nursing school or a seasoned veteran nurse, you'll appreciate this book.

- Ebi

CHAPTER 1

NURSING SCHOOL SUCKS

IT TOOK LIKE TEN DAYS TO GET MY final grades. One of the most stressful periods of my life. It was 2009, for Christ's sake; by then nearly every college in America utilized some sort of online classroom congregation that enabled instructors to post grades almost immediately. Not my school. I went to a community college nursing school that was stuck in the Stone Age—no Google Classroom, Moodle, or even Blackboard. I had to wait for my final grades to arrive in the mail.

The anxiety that was induced by such a stupid delay is basically nursing school in a nutshell: bullshit. The program, the professors, your clinical instructors, and even your classmates all try to shit on you in some fashion. A combination of lying, silly grudge-holding, and politicking makes an already difficult program even worse. Having to wait for my grades was simply the icing on the cake.

I remember maniacally checking for the mail every day after finals. We'd taken them the week after Thanksgiving, and now it was the second week of December. Chicago is typically frigid this time of year, and that combined with the stress of finals left me understandably on edge. As each day passed, my apprehension began to bottle. I was a pressurized mess of depression. In nursing school, no one has any idea how well they're doing. You can complete a test feeling confident and later find out you failed, and vice versa. Grades are truly a guessing game.

The envelope finally arrived. It was late in the afternoon and I had just completed a shift at my friend's video game store. Work provided plenty of distraction for me to temporarily stop obsessing. I walked into my kitchen, saw the envelope on the dining table, and took it upstairs—I wanted to be somewhere safe when I saw my grades. Using a blade, I cut the end of the envelope open and pulled out the contents. There were two pieces of paper, both tri-folded. I opened the top one. My calculated grade for Medical-Surgical Nursing II was displayed in large print.

Score: 83. I passed. Med-Surg is no easy task; it's a cluster of pathophysiology intertwined with health assessment and pharmacology. I took a deep sigh and, still staring at the number, absorbed the moment of relief. Then I tossed the paper to the side and picked up the one for Psych Nursing. It's just what it sounds like—a psychology class with nursing integration. Score: 79.3. My heart dropped. A score of 80 for the course was considered passing at my nursing school. This couldn't be right. Was this rounded incorrectly? Did I miss a quiz or assignment? Something had to give, because I did relatively well throughout the semester.

My professor's phone number was at the bottom of the letter, beneath her signature.

I spared no minute. I was fuming with anger and simultaneously in disbelief. I refused to accept that I would have to repeat the semester because of such a narrow margin. I listened to the loud ringing of the call through speakerphone until my professor answered, "Yes, hello?"

My emotions were taking over. I needed answers, something to explain this simply impossible grade. My voice cracked and I stuttered a bit. "Prof... professor?"

There was silence on the other end for what felt like an eternity. "Jaison, is that you?" Through my crackled mumble and the sniffling of my nose, she was able to identify me.

She continued on, "Jaison, I am so sorry. I went through every quiz, exam, and homework assignment to try to find the points you needed to get you to 79.5 so I can round you up to 80, but there was nothing and I just couldn't justify giving it to you."

I went into one of those heightened emotional states where everything goes white and all you hear is ringing—like being in the proximity of an explosion, except this was an emotional blast. My pride took a backseat and I began to beg, "Please. Please, professor. You can't do this to me."

My professor cut me off. "You did this to yourself. Just reapply to nursing school and take my class again. Enjoy the rest of your break." Click. She hung up before I could respond. She was done explaining herself and had no interest in consoling me. And I'd always thought I was her favorite student.

During the semester I was doing relatively well overall, so failing one class and barely passing another came to me as somewhat of a shock. There was a reasonable explanation, though, and I knew it.

Three weeks prior—a week before Thanksgiving—I was invited to a bachelor party and thoroughly enjoyed myself. My friends and I partied at someone's place and then made our way to the clubs in the cold Chicago night.

This was the height of the H1N1 virus, or swine flu, as the media called it. In nursing school, flu vaccines were required for clinical, but my half-assed nursing school didn't enforce it. Of course I was too lazy to go to Walgreens to get one. A flu outbreak, mixed with people in close contact at a club, is a recipe for disaster. I indulged.

The Monday of Thanksgiving week, I recall sitting in class and feeling a little off. I didn't think much of it because I had such a raunchy Saturday night; I assumed I was still hung over or catching a cold. I sat through all of class and slowly deteriorated throughout the day. Nearly six hours later, I was ready to go home. When Medical-Surgical II class ended, I was walking out and my professor, Professor Kristie, called me to her desk and asked me to meet her at her office. Nursing school is about bullshit, don't forget that.

I went to her office and waited by her door. A few minutes passed and I saw her walking down the hallway. She was overweight, a smoker, and always eating snacks. She huffed and puffed her way towards me and told me to open her office door and take a seat. I walked in and took my seat and she said she was going to grab someone else and to hang on one second. This is like the requisite of firing someone—you know, you go and get a witness, or backup, or whatever, just so there's someone else there to observe how the bad news is received.

Professor Kristie returned with her colleague and friend, the professor of Maternity Nursing, or "Mother/Baby," as everyone called it. Her name was Professor Crosby. She was a doctor, so students called her Professor or Doctor interchangeably. She appeared to be Professor Kristie's crony by the way you'd see them hang out a lot before and after lectures. Now they both walked in and stood over me. Professor Kristie asked me about clinical the week prior and how it went. I told her everyone was fine and inquired if there was a problem. She raised her eyebrows. "Yes, there was a problem, care to tell us what it was?" I was befuddled. I honestly didn't know of any problem. I shrugged my shoulders and told her that I wasn't feeling well and we needed to get to the point. She elaborated—and mind you, this is something that could get you expelled—"The clinical instructor told us that you administered morphine intravenously to a patient."

Nursing school is about bullshit.

I defended myself. "I didn't administer anything to anyone." During clinicals, students are allowed to pass oral medication under the supervision of a precepting nurse or instructor. During our nursing program, no IV medications are to be administered, and no narcotics of any kind. Morphine was a narcotic, and I was being accused of giving it IV. I recalled the event in question and gave her the truth. "The patient's nurse gave it, I was just there to observe. The nurse drew up the morphine and physically administered it. I was just an accessory."

Professor Kristie wasn't there, and she refused to expand on the allegation. She then laid down her punishment: "You are going to get the minimum passing grade for the clinical portion of this course, which is an 80%." This was unfair, because my clinical average was somewhere around 93% at the time, and I hadn't missed any clinicals. No proof, no evidence, no justice—it was my truth versus her claim, and I received my sentence. Professor Crosby nodded in agreement the whole time. I didn't fight it, I just informed both professors that I felt really sick and needed to go home. Coincidentally, I would have clinicals the next day with Professor Kristie. It was the last of the semester. I went home and went to bed early in the evening. I was sick emotionally and physically.

The next morning, I woke up at about 4 a.m. My head was spinning and I was running a fever. I was incredibly weak and nauseous. I texted one of my classmates for Professor Kristie's number, then immediately texted her and let her know I was miserably sick and might go to the hospital. She was already up because we had to be at our clinical site at 6 a.m. I couldn't read much of her reaction via text, but she kept her responses very brief. I bet she thought I was faking the whole thing. We are allowed to miss one clinical day the whole semester, so technically I didn't need to be there, but I wasn't sure what my standing was since my grade for clinical was already declared the minimum.

My mom took me to the doctor around 10 a.m. and they performed a swab test deep into my nasal sinus passage. The swab was tested on-site and confirmed to be swine flu. I got it from the club on Saturday night, I am 100% sure of it. My doctor prescribed me Tamiflu and I started it that day.

I called Professor Kristie later that day and we had a nice little chat about my future in the nursing program. She was concerned I would not be well enough for finals next week and suggested I take an "incomplete" for the courses since it was too late in the semester to withdraw. It was a Tuesday, and finals were Wednesday and Thursday the next week, with optional review sessions on that Monday and Tuesday. I guaranteed her that I would be ready for finals. She then hit me with a small demand—that I get a doctor's note for clearance to return to class. I inquired about my situation being classified as a medical emergency and whether there was any way I could take the finals a few days late. She defiantly informed me that "under no circumstance will any student be taking the finals before or after anyone else."

I returned home from my doctor's office and began my road to recovery. I had about five or six days to get it together. I used to do this trick whenever I got sick with a bad cold or flu: I would drink a bottle of water an hour while I was awake and keep from doing anything strenuous. Meaning, I would lie around and nap or play videogames all day. The idea here was to just urinate nonstop and make whatever virus I had run its course faster. I always believed it to work, but I won't argue with those who claim that every successful attempt of mine was a fluke. I was slamming down waters all week and into the weekend. My girlfriend at the time stopped by one time for a few minutes and dropped off a day's worth of Thanksgiving dinner. I kept myself well-nourished and over-hydrated.

By Friday, there wasn't much improvement. I was still miserable and my fever wouldn't go down. I was becoming increasingly anxious that I wouldn't be ready for finals. Still, I called my doctor and told him I was feeling "okay" and wanted to see him Monday to receive my note for clearance. I'd rather he deny me than never to have tried. As Saturday rolled around, I continued my water-drinking regimen and started to feel a little better. I was less weak, that's for sure. While in my bedroom, I started jogging in place to increase my heart rate and develop a sweat. I needed as much water going out as going in. I was determined to get this virus to run its course as fast as possible. Drinking, sweating, peeing, repeat. I think I took three or four showers that day. I fell asleep around seven that evening and slept till ten on Sunday—a full fifteen hours.

When I woke up, I was still exhausted and feverish and I decided it was probably time to evaluate my new one-year plan. I could take a pair of "incompletes" for my courses and try again the next year. It would be a medically-related reason for leaving nursing school right before finals, but it would be justified. I accepted defeat and decided my whole life was now going to be a year late. Depressed, I continued to drink water like a madman throughout Sunday and into the evening.

I slept another fifteen hours and got dressed for my doctor's appointment on Monday. I was feeling pretty good. It helped that the weather was warm and the sun was shining. I got to the doctor's office and a nurse took my vital signs. Everything was normal. My fever was gone. I still felt weak and miserable, but I hid it as best as I could. My doctor looked at me and said, "Okay, what do you need from me?"

I told him how badly I needed a note that would allow me to return to class and take finals. He agreed, but under some terms: "You have to wear a mask, don't cough, and don't interact with anyone. Take your finals and go home." Sounded like a deal to me.

Since I had my note in hand, I figured I could attend the last review session the next day. I'd been so incapacitated the whole past week, I hadn't studied one bit for two finals that were in control of my life's course. I continued to drink water and pee all day for the rest of Monday. On Tuesday, I still felt miserable. I could feel I was running a fever again, but I didn't bother to actually check—it would've stressed me out too much, and I already had too many problems on my plate. I got ready and headed to the finals review session wrapped up in a hoodie and a medical mask. I had everything tight because I didn't want to risk getting anyone sick or getting more sick myself.

I walked into the lecture hall that was hosting the review. Standing in front of the whole class was Professor Kristie. She turned to look at me in the doorway after seeing the surprised reactions of my classmates. "Nope," she said. "You can't be here. I need a note." I walked towards her, and she took a few steps back and placed her hand over her mouth and nose. I pulled the note out my back pocket and placed it on desk that sat between us on the staging area of the lecture all. Through my mask I muffled, "Right there. I am clear to be here and I am clear for finals." I looked around the lecture hall for a seat that wasn't too close to anyone. Professor Kristie peered at the note on the desk, and without touching it she pointed to a random desk near the exit and ordered, "You don't sit near anyone. Take that desk and set up in the corner. If you have a question, write it down. Please don't talk. Thanks." Treat me like an animal, I guess. Fuck nursing school.

I saw through the review and absorbed all of the information I could. It wasn't easy with a pounding headache and that general uncomfortable feeling. I was trying to process months of information for an exam I probably wasn't ready for. I'd been doing fairly well throughout the semester, though, so I could get a 75 or 80 on the final exam and still pass the course.

This was just for Medical-Surgical Nursing II, of course. I'd missed the review for Psych Nursing the day before. I didn't worry too much about that class, though; I was doing really well there.

I did the best I could at taking notes and trying to identify what was going to be on the final. The review lecture helped, people asked some good questions, including a few about subjects I never even knew we covered. Great. I went home and spent the rest of the evening studying for the first final I'd take the next day: Psych.

I woke up feeling like absolute shit, nearly as bad as the first day I had the swine flu. This final was not going to go well. I dragged myself out of bed, got ready, and headed to school. I grabbed my desk and set up camp away from all of the other students and faced the wall. My professor and her proctor handed out the exams. My professor stopped at my desk and said, "I'm surprised you made it. Everyone in the department was expecting you to take the 'incomplete.' You know, if you don't pass, you have a long road ahead of you."

This is nursing school. Professors want to see you crash and burn. They live for it. Especially if you're one of the well-known, respected students. It's such a weird dynamic. It's almost as if the professors' job is to weed out not only students that would make bad nurses, but an additional chunk of them—just to be safe.

I started my final with the extra dose of stress that my professor just fed me. As I navigated through the final, all things considered, I felt alright about it. Psych Nursing was something I understood confidently, and my grades and work ethic throughout the semester supported that claim.

The exam was a hundred questions, many of which I had seen on prior quizzes. This was a good test, I'd take it. I felt good. I was one of the first ones to complete it, too. I bounced out of there and went home to spend the rest of the day in bed.

I was in no shape for the next final. It was like the swine flu got its second wind or something. Typically, this kind of virus can take two to three weeks to recover from, and here I was trying to take finals only a week after diagnosis and treatment. I headed into my Medical-Surgical Nursing II final anyway. This final required real critical thinking skills and a strong foundation of knowledge. It was the same deal as during the review session—I walked into the room and my professor pointed me to the corner, berated me for being there, and handed me my exam. It's wild how professors will be your friend all semester and then turn on you for something out of your control.

Remember, I'd missed the Psych review and I didn't spend much time studying for the final in the days leading up to it. Let's also not forget I didn't study at all during those first six days I was sick. Psych was my confidence class, and I was trucking on through the semester. But I'd really needed to focus on Medical-Surgical Nursing II.

Once I laid eyes on the exam, I knew I was done for. None of the questions looked familiar, and I couldn't think of any answers through the fogginess in my mind and the creeping fever. My body was aching and shaking with the chills. Yup, I was bombing this test. I was hoping to get just enough correct to pass the class. All I needed on this final was a 72. The final carried some heavy final grade percentage, but my quiz and homework grades were relatively high. This time, I was one of the last students to complete the exam. I sat up from my seat and handed the exam in to my professor. She looked at me and rolled her eyes. I guess she knew I bombed it? I never bothered to ask.

My nursing program was really wonky. You weren't allowed to review any of your exams or quizzes after finals, and final grade calculations were held in secrecy. The grade you calculated on your own was never the grade you actually received. I remember hearing my professor say once, "Sometimes we have to push some students over," in response to my inquiry about such high-level secrecy with grades.

Circling back to that miserable day I received my grades, when I realized that everything was a done deal and I'd officially failed the class I was certain I'd pass. The next step in my program was to basically beg to be reinstated for the next year, which would be fall 2010. The process required that I have a phone call with the director of the nursing program and inform them that I planned to reapply. Once my phone call was acknowledged by the director, I would be given a meeting date. This meeting would consist of me showing up with a typed letter that explained my game plan, everything I would do differently to ensure success the next time around. I would present my plan to the director and three professors in a format resembling *American Idol*. Yes, these people would judge my plan and provide their opinions and feedback, and then I would find out whether I'd get the golden ticket into the nursing program (again!).

I completed my phone call with the director three days after receiving my failure letter. The director of my nursing program was a wonderful lady. She was compassionate and considerate and seemed to really sympathize with the students as they navigated the stressors of nursing school. On the phone, she expressed shock that I didn't pass one of my classes and ensured me that everything was going to be okay. She then said that she had confidence in my ability to impress at the return interview. She gave me a date for the interview and wished me luck.

While drafting my letter of intent to return to the nursing program, I was conflicted. Did I want to go through this again? Was this even the career for me? Was swine flu a blessing in disguise, the hint I needed to change course? These are questions nursing students ask themselves every day. Many take the exit and never return. I don't blame them. The unreasonable difficulty of the program and lack of empathy from the professors can turn the most weathered-skinned students away. On top of those things considered, what would my letter even say? I had to provide the "panel of judges" a game plan that would instill the confidence required to give me another chance. I always studied plenty and I was an ideal student; I couldn't just say that I planned to be happy and healthy the next time finals rolled around. I just drafted up the bullshit they wanted to hear—"I'll study more and put more hours in the clinical lab and review the material more often," whatever.

The day of my meeting arrived. It was in the middle of the week before Christmas and a week after grades arrived. I didn't have much time to think before I hastily decided to take the meeting. I dressed up like it was a job interview: freshly pressed pants, a dress shirt, and the shoes to match. I had my declaration prepared and printed several copies, as there was no clarification as to how many I should bring.

My stress level was at an all-time high. I couldn't even eat that day. I was nearly three weeks post-swine flu and I still wasn't feeling completely well. I had no Plan B. If the director and her goons rejected my proposal, I'd be done—I'd just find a trade or union job and go that route.

I made my way through the college buildings toward the nursing department. In the lounge area, I saw a few other students. They were the others who had failed and were here for their own interviews. There's a shame attached with failing, so when grades come out, you hear about all the people who passed and are out celebrating. Those who fail stay quiet. It's embarrassing to tell people you didn't pass, especially when there's an expectation that you'll be just fine. I'm sure we were all in the same boat of depression.

I headed to the nursing department office area to check in. I said hello to the clerk and she instructed me to wait in the lounge area for someone to come get me when it was my turn. The air was dense and the aura was tense. It was the same feeling you have when you walk into someone's wake—you kind of acknowledge people with that half smile. Really no conversation, just enough shrugging to establish the reason you're all here. One classmate of mine was sobbing in the back of the lounge. I don't know if she'd had her turn already and was told she wasn't coming back, or if she was still waiting but feeling overwhelmed by this deliberately stressful process.

I picked a chair and sat by myself. Everyone was by themselves. Some were listening to their iPods, others texting, I sat staring blankly at the bulletin board in front of me. Posted were events of weeks past. Nothing posted for the future. This was winter break, so there were no students walking the halls. You'd see the occasional custodian walk by as he received orders from his walkie-talkie. It was eerie being in the building and waiting for your fate. For me, it was basically, "You're going to live, or you're going to die. Good luck."

Nursing was life or death for us students. Many of my classmates were from unfortunate upbringings and disadvantaged neighborhoods, and this program was their only way out. If they were rejected readmission into nursing school, their lives were essentially over. If I didn't get back into in the program, my life would mostly be over too. Well, my parents would've supported me enough to get me back on my feet and help me head into a new direction. Only problem? I didn't have a back-up plan, like most of my classmates. It was boom or bust.

I could hear the tapping of someone's shoes from down the hallway. Someone was coming from the direction of the nursing department. All the students in the lounge looked up. It was the nursing secretary, come to gather her next victim. She smiled and called a name. The student acknowledged and the secretary gestured him to follow. I kept looking down the hallway to see if any students were returning from their meetings, but no one ever came back this way. It appeared they were leaving through a door on the opposite end of the building.

Every thirty minutes or so, the secretary would come and grab someone. Same tapping, same smile, same gesture—she was a robot. Our emotions were high while the administrators were dead cold. This was clockwork for them. They did this every semester. As I waited patiently for my turn, the student sobbing calmed down a bit. No one asked her if she was okay, no one spoke to each other in that lounge. We all remembered in the back of our minds that not everyone was getting back into nursing school. I know this sounds awful, but the more of an emotional wreck this girl was, the better chances I had at securing my spot. I needed to only worry about me.

I had an appointment, and I waited over ninety minutes past the appointed time. I think the director and her instructors took a lunch at some point, because I remember waiting around and not really seeing any activity.

Once again, I heard the secretary make her way back to the lounge. Somehow I knew it was my turn. She walked in and said, "Jaison, they're ready to see you now."

I took a deep breath and gathered my belongings. My hands were shaking and I was a nervous wreck. I walked behind the secretary as she tried to make small talk with me. "Jaison, I'm surprised you're in the position to reapply. What happened?" I shrugged my shoulders and let out a big sigh. "It was a collection of things, I don't know." This wasn't something I wanted to get into during the one-minute walk to the department, though it did feel like an eternity.

She escorted me into the department and told me to take a seat on a cold steel chair. This was the last thing I needed before the meeting of my life—to be cold and uncomfortable. Granted, the college was empty, but I would have hoped they still ran the furnace for the few administrators who were sticking around. My knees were shaking; I was now both cold and nervous. I was so glad I opted not to eat breakfast; otherwise I would have thrown it up several times by now. I sat staring at this one door knowing that on the other side were the director and her professors.

The door suddenly opened and the director stood in the doorway saying, "Jaison, what a pleasant surprise. We are ready to see you now." I gathered my belongings again, shaking, cold, nervous, sick to my stomach. I wanted to cry now. I walked in. Facing me was a long table with four seats occupied by the professor of Maternity Nursing, Dr. Crosby; the professor of first year Medical-Surgical Nursing, Professor Haley (I passed her class the year before with some issues); the head of the nursing clinical laboratory, Professor Mary; and of course, the director of the program, Donna.

Professor Haley always gave me trouble, and for no reason. Once upon a time, when I first got accepted to nursing school, the students were invited to an open house to meet our classmates and professors. It wasn't a mandatory event. It was a nice informal gathering before orientation, just to meet people and exchange numbers and such. I recall it being held on a hot summer morning. Everyone wore regular summer clothes. I was in shorts and a T-shirt. I made my way through each station at the event, introducing myself to alumni, current students, and faculty. I made my way to Professor Haley and introduced myself with, "Hi, I'm Jaison. I'll be in the nursing program this fall." She sized me up and down and said, "I guess they let anyone in now, huh." I nervously laughed, not sure if she was joking. She then continued, "If you want to make it in the program, you're going to have to dress a little more respectful and get rid of your earrings." My ears were pierced at the time. I didn't think it was going to be an issue during class, though I was well aware of the jewelry rule for clinicals—you weren't allowed to have any, and I get it, that's okay—so I politely rebutted, "I don't have a problem removing them for clinicals, and they're just earrings." She rolled her eyes at me. "I know you won't have a problem with that, but I suggest you also keep them at home during class. Especially my class." Shoulder-motherfucking-shrugging emoji. I just shrugged so hard, I had nothing else to respond with. Needless to say, I kept my earrings off her whole course. It is sad how important the perception of power is to some of these professors. It was a non-issue for me; I didn't care about my earrings as much as she thought I did.

I realized the true extent of her dislike for me during the end of my semester with her. In your first year of nursing school, you learn how to clean patients, perform head-to-toe assessments, and take vital signs. To ensure you perform these skills safely and effectively, you have to take this stressful exam called the clinical return demonstration. You perform all these processes with a mannequin while the professor of the clinical laboratory and your professor for Medical-Surgical Nursing observe and grade. The return demonstrations were scheduled for a Monday and I remember staying late in the lab on the Friday before, to practice my skills for the exam. I was confident I was going to knock the test out of the park. It was all repetition—if you practiced enough, you would pass this test. But of course, along with all the other exams and nuances in nursing school, the professors made sure you were stressed about this. After spending some hours after class in the lab, I headed out and passed by Professor Haley's office. She was grading papers with her door open. As I walked by and glanced inside, she made eye contact with me. I waved and said, "See you Monday." I kept walking and I heard her voice drift into the hallway. "You better be ready for the return demonstrations." I turned and peeked my head back into her doorway. "Yeah, 8 a.m., I'll see you there. I'm good to go." She smiled and corrected me, "8:30 a.m. The return demos begin 8:30 a.m. Get that rest, you don't have to come that early." I was confused, as I was certain it was at 8 a.m. "Are you sure it's 8:30 a.m.? I thought 8 a.m." She doubled down. "No, no. It is 8:30, see you then." I thanked her and went on my way to enjoy my weekend.

I did some light practicing of the return demo in my bedroom. I had it down pat. When Monday rolled around, I got ready and headed to campus. Luckily for me, it was only a ten-minute drive, so I never had to rush in the morning. As I walked through the nursing department, the hallways were noticeably quiet. It was around 8:15, and people usually hung around in the hallways until class started. I walked to the laboratory to take my spot for the return demonstration and opened the door. It was silent in there. Students were working on the mannequins as the professors observed and graded. The return demos had begun already, and I was late. I saw Professor Haley and hurried to her station. I was frantically trying to get my things in order, saying, "I'm sorry, you told me 8:30, so I figured I still had plenty of time." She scoffed at my apology. "You know the exams always begin 8 a.m. sharp. You know the rules. If you're late, you're not allowed to take the exam."

She tried to sabotage me! She had some nerve to lie outright about the time. I always felt like she had a target on me, and never knew why. Professor Mary was in charge of my station and walked in as I was trying to plead my case to Professor Haley. She said, "Oh, we're just beginning. It's okay, Jaison, get situated and we will begin." Professor Mary was always nice to students.

I performed my return demonstration and scored a perfect 100% under Professor Mary's scoring grid. Professor Haley scored me at 85%, citing that I wasn't very clear with hand-washing technique and other things. It was so trivial; she was just deducting points for its own sake. Nursing school professors like her hold grudges. They use every bit of their power to emotionally abuse you. Now I had the pleasure of dealing with Professor Haley again, as part of the panel that would decide whether or not I could re-enter nursing school. Holding this power over me was probably like cocaine to her.

I sat there in the director's office, sitting across from the panel of judges, and pulled out my useless game plan to read to them. It was just generic planning. I talked about studying more, paying better attention, and working fewer hours at my job. I also focused on my strengths: how I was a solid student and I was doing well before I became sick. The director understood and hung onto each word while Professor Mary, being the student advocate that she was, nodded in agreement.

Professor Haley took this opportunity to trash me. "What you did to pass the semester wasn't enough, and I don't think you possess the capacity to make the necessary changes. You are not fit for nursing."

I gestured vaguely. "I have been an ideal student up until the moment I became sick. I completed the whole first year nearly effortlessly. I was even tutoring other students on the pharmacology sections of your class, do you not remember?"

Professor Haley doubled down as she liked to do. "Just because you're good at math don't mean you'll make a good nurse."

Dr. Crosby chimed in, "Jaison, you are too autonomous, and that is dangerous for this line of work. Doctors don't appreciate that."

I felt backed into a corner, and besides, I learned years later that any doctor would appreciate a smart, autonomous nurse.

I don't know their process of collectively deciding which students were allowed back into the program and which were kicked to the curb. They continued to ask questions about why I failed and what I was going to do differently, and I kept repeating myself and redirecting their attention to my history as a successful student. The idea of a student tanking at the end of the semester due solely to an illness just wasn't fully registering with them. Once it was apparent that my answers were going to remain the same, and their questions weren't changing, Donna told me that the interview was over and they would contact me. As I was gathering my things, she informed me that there were only five spots for returning students, and more than twelve were vying for those spots. She wished me luck and showed me the door.

I walked out and the secretary had me sign some paperwork and put her hand on my shoulder. "I think you should be given another chance, you'd make a great nurse. You are so detail oriented." I thanked her and she showed me out, asking me to leave the opposite way of the lounge. I guess they didn't want me passing along the experience to the other students waiting. It didn't matter to me; I felt defeated.

I went home and began planning my next career. I had zero confidence that I was making it back into the program. The number of seats was limited and two of the panel didn't want me back in for unknown reasons. I believe it was simply a personality conflict and a fundamental discrimination against male nurses (plenty of that later). After searching online for some union jobs and city jobs, I gave up. I called my girlfriend and we went to have dinner downtown.

I decompressed during our drive into the city. We were going to one of my favorite restaurants (doesn't matter where, they're not sponsoring me). It was around 6:30 p.m., and my girlfriend and I had just found parking when my phone rang. It was an unknown number. I was skeptical of it being a telemarketer, but it was a Friday, and it was after hours anyway. I answered. The voice on the other end said, "Jaison, did I catch you at a bad time?" I was just making my way out of my car but immediately sat back inside and closed the door. My girlfriend did the same; she could read my face. I responded, "Yes, this is Jaison, who's this?" The voice laughed. "It's Donna, the director. How are you?" My heart beat out of my throat and I struggled to hold it together. Maybe she just wanted some more information? I responded briefly, "Yeah, I'm good, how are you?" Donna was uncomfortably joyful. "I am doing well. I want to share some news with you." Oh Lord Jesus Christ, the news is coming literally hours after I sat through the worst interview of my life. It must be bad, because you can more quickly decide no rather than yes—right? Donna continued, "I would like formally invite you back into the nursing program next fall. I know you are going to be one of the best nurses to walk across that stage." I held back tears, thanking her over and over again, and then we exchanged pleasantries and I told her I was turning my depression dinner into a celebration. I couldn't help but ask about the other professors, though. "It sounded like half the room didn't want me back... what was the deal?" She laughed. "I have the final say. We need more male nurses in this industry. We need more male nurses like you. Some people are too old-fashioned to get that. I know you'll make me proud."

It had certainly been a rollercoaster ride of a couple weeks, but I was back in the nursing program. The only problem was that I had to wait until the following fall. I had the spring semester free to do as I pleased. When the new semester began, I took a class I didn't need; I just wanted to be enrolled in something to keep access to the college. Professor Mary told me that I could use the nursing lab anytime during the semester. I didn't take her words lightly; I was there twice a week for two hours a day. I reviewed quiz questions and exam questions, read the material for future classes, and more. I basically taught myself the semester of nursing the students were currently in—I wanted to be over-prepared. I also reviewed all of the Psych Nursing stuff I would have to repeat the coming fall.

When the fall semester rolled around, I enrolled only in the course I had to repeat. I was stone cold, stone-faced, total Mamba Mentality, Kobe-zoned out the whole semester. I was still so angry with how the faculty treated me. With that chip on my shoulder, I had no friends—and I certainly wasn't friendly with the faculty. But I rocked every Psych quiz and exam. I was scoring 95% or higher on everything that was thrown in my direction. When finals were on the horizon again, I was happy and healthy. I rocked them and finished with a 94% as my final grade in Psych Nursing. Some even accused me of having the answers to all the quizzes and exams. Well, I did, it was all the same shit from the year before. I had studied it to death in the lab.

When the fall semester ended, I received some surprising news: Donna was fired. I was quite shocked; I didn't know what to make of it. When the spring semester began, there was news that she had accepted a position as director of another nursing school under the same organization. Rumors were spreading, and the accepted story was that she was in fact fired, and threatened to sue, and was immediately rehired at that other nursing school. I never found out the truth.

We weren't without a director for long. Professor Haley was promoted shortly after spring classes began. Exactly what I needed, my sworn enemy (and for no reason) was in charge of everyone and everything. She wasn't teaching any courses I needed in my final semester, thankfully. My only concern was Dr. Crosby's Maternity Nursing course (Mother/Baby, that is).

I tried to keep a low-profile in Mother/Baby, but Dr. Crosby would pick on me so much. She would call on me for deliberately difficult questions and make me feel like shit when I didn't have the answers. I'd look around the classroom and see that no one else had them either. I never retaliated; I always made sure to keep my cool. I was in no position to feud with anyone. I was a loner and my greatest ally was gone.

There was one incident where Dr. Crosby and I bickered over the difference between osmosis and diffusion. She had mixed the two up and I politely corrected her before mass confusion ensued, and she ripped me apart. She said things like, "Wait until you become a doctor before you start correcting me." Okay, sure, I wanted no issues. I left the situation alone and carried on. She took a lot of pride in being a doctor and defended the role heavily; in fact, it was odd how defensive she would get sometimes. But it was also important to note she would make mindless errors that didn't reflect a medical school education. I chalked it up to old age. A year later, Dr. Crosby would be indicted on charges of theft to government property. Turned out she had falsified her doctoral degree and transcripts and was teaching as a doctor and receiving doctor's pay. She fled out West. What a fucking bum. That nursing school continued to be a shit show even after I left.

Anyway, because I had spent so much time in the nursing lab the year before (during my semester break), I breezed through the final lap of nursing school. As my final act of defiance, I skipped the pinning ceremony and graduation. Nurses know how important pinning ceremony is. For those out of the loop, it's a symbolic ceremony performed by nursing schools to welcome the graduating class into the nursing profession. There is an actual pin, or badge, that is fastened onto the new graduate's garment by the faculty. (It's more common now to be "pinned" by a family member or a close friend.) Students then recite the Florence Nightingale pledge. It's a big deal. Everyone talks about the pinning ceremony. Students wear their best outfits and celebrate with fancy dinners afterward. And I skipped it. I was glad I did, and sitting here ten years later, I'd make that decision again.

Professor Haley called me a few days after the pinning ceremony and told me it was disrespectful that I chose to skip it. I told her I was skipping graduation as well and to take a hike. We hung up on each other.

I picked up my diploma a few weeks later. I walked past the same lounge near the nursing department and saw the sad faces of some classmates of mine. They were here for that shitty pride-stripping process of begging your way back into nursing school. I wanted to stop by and give some words of encouragement, but fuck them. It wasn't anything personal. It was just that I wanted nothing to do with this school ever again.

Nearly every nursing student will agree that nursing school is very difficult. The programs are typically fast-tracked. You are taking only two classes a semester, but both entail long class times and day-long clinicals in between (upwards of twelve hours), and various assignments take up your free days. Before you know it, two classes take up nearly sixty hours between Monday and Friday. Studying on Sunday helps a lot, and leaving Saturday as your decompression day will do wonders for the mind.

You have to manage your time well. Identify your strengths and weaknesses as a student and build off that knowledge. Some people have to study a lot, while others read material once and know it forever. While in nursing school, I was working about twenty to thirty hours a week. For me, it was doable, while for some of my classmates, they had to quit their jobs and focus 100% on nursing. For the record, not working is recommended.

You have to put in the time to study the questions and understand the material. You'll be surprised to see how much easier quizzes and exams can be when you have a good foundation of knowledge, as some questions will help you answer others.

In my nursing program, no one wanted to help each other. There were some small groups and cliques that stuck together, but generally, everyone was on their own. If someone is willing to help you, accept it, but don't get bent out of shape if you feel like you are treading water alone. Nursing school admissions are very competitive, and a lot of that sentiment carries into the program itself. Students forget that the job market is wide open—there will always be more positions than nurses applying. Everyone who graduates, I assure you, will find a job.

CHAPTER 2

DEALING WITH EXIT EXAMS AND THE NCLEX

I **THINK EVERY NURSING SCHOOL HAS AN EXIT EXAM—AND** if yours didn't, you better double-check the validity of your degree. The exit exam exists because nursing schools need as many graduates as possible to pass the NCLEX (Nursing Council Licensure Examination) on their first try. They boast their passing rates to attract students. Certain states also require nursing school to maintain a certain percentage of NCLEX "passers" (governing bodies have to ensure nursing schools are doing their job, right?). In many nursing schools, if you don't pass the exit exam, they don't sign off on you taking the NCLEX. This practice helps lower their NCLEX fail rate. The problem with these exit exams, though, is that they are ridiculously difficult and don't represent the NCLEX very well. Many schools utilize the HESI (Health Education Systems Incorporated) exam. Not only is the HESI exam really hard, but it fails to be a proper measuring tool for schools to determine whether students will pass the NCLEX. Many students who fail the HESI are still capable of passing the NCLEX.

Practice makes perfect. Do practice exam questions any spare moment you have. You can never do enough. Though nursing is a vast spectrum, there are a finite number of questions that can be asked for the NCLEX. The NCLEX only wants to make sure you are a safe practicing nurse, one that is ready to learn to be a real nurse in the field.

When I had my semester off from nursing school, I took thorough advantage of Professor Mary's offer of access to the lab. As you may recall, I studied the material from the classes that I would've been taking had I not failed Psych Nursing, so that I would be up to speed and ahead when I actually enrolled in those classes. But I didn't just keep myself busy with mundane phantom homework assignments and quizzes. I was also practicing for the NCLEX two hours a day twice a week.

Our nursing lab had nearly every NCLEX resource a student could ask for. The one I utilized the most was this cheap computer program called the NCLEX 3500. It originally came out in 2004, with various updates since then. The program is 3,500 multiple-choice questions. You select a category and the number of questions you want to deal with. I would get through about a hundred questions in two hours when I first started using it. If you get a question right, you move on. If you get a question wrong, rationales are provided. I would read the rationale, and then move on. By the end of the semester, I was breezing through almost three hundred questions a session. I understood and memorized the rationales to 3,500 NCLEX questions. I was a man possessed.

If doing seemingly mindless multiple-choice tests for hours on end isn't your thing, there are tons of other resources. You could do anything from the Saunders or Lippincott libraries. The point is, practice and repetition are effective in passing the NCLEX. It truly is that simple.

What about those NCLEX review courses? Yeah, I took one. I took probably one of the best ones anyone can offer. This Filipino nurse (we'll call her Lola) would teach a

NCLEX review course at a Filipino community center on the North Side of Chicago. I don't want to give away too many details about her, because her method was sketchy. The class took place the first week of a month, Monday through Friday, from 9 a.m. to 2 p.m. There were about forty people in attendance and we would spend hours taking practice NCLEX exams and going over all of the questions we answered incorrectly. It was basically the NCLEX 3500, except in person. This was an effective course if you were a face-to-face, hands-on type of learner.

Nurse Lola would offer you half your money back if you failed the NCLEX and allow you to retake her course for free. It was a pretty sweet deal if you think about it. I think it was around $250 to take her course at the time.

Here's the kicker, though. On the final day of her course, she asked everyone to memorize one question from the NCLEX and immediately email it to her afterwards. I looked around the room and tried to digest the reactions to that request. Some people smiled and were on board, a few didn't pay any attention, and others clearly weren't going to do it. I gathered that about ten people were going to go through with her request. Lola had been doing this course for years, but it wasn't until this moment that I realized that all the practice exams we'd been doing were probably sourced from former attendees who had given her questions from the NCLEX. So I knew I was going to pass the NCLEX. I'd basically taken the equivalent of ten NCLEX exams over the past five days. All the questions had to have come from past attendees. This was gold... and probably illegal too. Yeah, it was 100% illegal.

Was I going to take part in these shenanigans? Only time would tell. By the completion of Lola's NCLEX course, my date with the NCLEX was about three weeks away. My objective was for the NCLEX to be a one-night-stand deal, no plans for a second date.

Weeks prior—around the time I graduated—I had applied for the NCLEX exam. A lot of students like to take the NCLEX as soon as they graduate, so spaces fill up quick. I graduated in May and scheduled my NCLEX for the end of June. I believe it was the first week of June I took Lola's course, so everything kind of lined up nicely for me.

When you apply, you get to select a testing location. Naturally I chose the one closest to my home. It was downtown, about a forty-minute drive for me in the morning. Anything can happen on a relatively long commute like that. It is what it is. My only suggestion is to arrive very early and relax before the exam starts. Avoid distractions or any bad vibes the days leading up to the exam and the morning of the exam. I scheduled my NCLEX for 10 a.m. because it was around the same time of day I'd been doing all my NCLEX 3500 practice questions, and right in the middle of Lola's NCLEX course. My mind was already trained to tackle questions at that hour. I recommend you do the same—there is research that supports improved test scores for those who take exams at the same time they study.

About a week before the exam, I cleaned up my diet. I cut out all processed foods and simple carbohydrates and stuck to a diet that was rich in protein, complex carbs, and fiber. I avoided alcohol and drank only water. It was difficult for me because I almost always partied on weekends, and I had really let loose after graduation. I also like to indulge in a can of pop every few days, so refraining from that was difficult too. I was going to the gym pretty regularly already, but to optimize my mental clarity, I ramped up my gym attendance. I was going every day and staying twice as long.

Heading into the NCLEX, I was feeling great. I stayed off social media and didn't tell anyone when I was going to take the test. I didn't want anyone to accidentally say something negative to me and bring me down. There are some serious haters out there that low-key want to see you fail. Don't give anyone the chance to even come with that vibe.

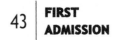

Some students make the mistake of cramming during the week leading up to the exam. Here's the deal: If you don't know it now, you're not going to master it a week before the test. You'll end up fumbling your information and confusing fundamental concepts on test day. The franticness of cram sessions isn't healthy for the mind when taking an exam that will make or break your career.

The night before the exam, I made sure to rest well. I went to bed early, I avoided watching anything stressful, and I maintained my distance from social media. I researched my route to the testing center to make sure I was prepared for the time it would take in morning traffic. My plan was to arrive about forty-five minutes early so I could relax and decompress in the waiting area.

The morning of the test I felt well rested but amped with adrenaline. Even with all the dieting, exercise, and mental preparations, I still woke up a nervous wreck. Aside from being one of the most important exams you'll ever take, there's another underlying factor that intensifies the stress: the unknown. The NCLEX has no set number of questions. You will answer at least 75 questions or up to 265. The test gauges your knowledge as a new graduate nurse and actively decides as you go along whether you need to answer more questions, or enough is enough.

You might answer seventy-five questions and then fail the NCLEX... or pass it with flying colors. Or you might answer almost three hundred questions, and again the result may just as well be passing as failing.

The anxiety of knowing that the test may end at any time is very real. Unless you have a clear grasp of the covered material, your presumed result can feel like a flip of the coin. Did you pass, did you fail? You'll have to just wait until the official results.

Anyway, back to the morning of the NCLEX. Traffic was forgiving that day, and I arrived at the test site about an hour ahead of time. I found parking and walked around the block once to burn off some energy. Downtown Chicago has some really beautiful views during the summer, and there are lots of people walking around. It was such a relaxer, I could have easily done four more laps. I was careful though—it was a warm June day and I didn't want to show up sweaty. I entered the office building and checked in at the front desk, then took the elevator up to testing facility. Upon my arrival on the sixth floor, I was met with a reception area where some people were sitting around. One girl slouched on the end of a couch, her eyes puffy and red, staring into the distance. Actually, there was a random potted fern in her line of sight, but she looked glazed enough for me to assume that wasn't her focus. I walked over to the reception desk and checked in. Two forms of ID—I brought my state ID and passport. The state wants to make sure that it is YOU taking this NCLEX. I wouldn't try to do otherwise. If you somehow were to scam a way into having someone else take the test for you, you are only hurting yourself and every future patient you encounter. Not worth it.

I checked in and was finger-printed as well. The receptionist told me I was early and to relax in the lobby with the others and check back in about a half hour. I made my way back to the lobby and looked at all the faces around me. I didn't recognize anyone, which was good. You don't want any added pressure on a day like this. The one girl who seemed to be having a bad day looked up at me and took a deep breath. "Are taking the NCLEX?" I sat down across from her with a feeling of where this was going just based on how she looked. I answered, "Yeah, my appointment is 10 a.m. Just kind of chilling out before it's my time." She sniffled a bit. "Two hundred thirty-five questions and it shut off for me. Not one looked familiar. I totally guessed my way through. I know I'll have to take this again." Okay, thanks for bringing me down, bitch. I didn't know how to respond, so I said, "I'm sorry, hopefully it's not as bad as you think." She wiped her eyes, her frustration apparent on her face. "I'm just waiting for my friend to pick me up so we can go drinking." No judging here, she was already a nurse in my eyes—drinking at odd hours and shit. More on that later. "Hey, you never know. Just check the results in two days, and hopefully you'll have happy reasons to drink."

The girl answered her vibrating phone and made her way out after wishing me luck. Two hundred thirty-five questions is a lot; I would guess she failed, but honestly, chances were fifty-fifty. As the minutes passed, I watched other potential exam-takers make their way out of the lobby. Before I knew it, it was 9:55. Time to go. I made my way back to the receptionist, who checked my identity again. I had to check all of my belongings into a locker before making my way into the testing area. You are more than welcome to access your locker and check your phone and belongings during the test, and you can use the restroom as needed as well. You do have to check in and out with the receptionist and confirm your identity each time you leave your testing station. This is serious stuff, and the exam is not to be taken lightly.

It was now or never for me. I'd done everything I could to prepare for the exam. Whatever the outcome following today, it was my fate. The test area was tightly observed by a proctor who walked up and down between stations, tending to anyone who had a question or concern. The proctor showed me to my station, handed me my headphones, and told me to raise my hand when I was complete with the test or if I needed anything. Click start whenever you are ready.

The first question appeared on the screen. It was a subject matter I had never studied or heard of before. I remember thinking, "This sounds like something a veteran nurse should know, we didn't learn this." After reading through the possible answers, I had no idea which direction to take this question. I didn't even have an educated guess. I picked option C, because fuck it. Before submitting my answer, I sat and thought about what I had gotten myself into. I really hoped I wouldn't have to endure the next 265 or however many questions feeling this disappointment in myself. I clicked onto the next question.

Question number two rolled in and it was something I had seen before. About four words into the question, I mouthed, "I know this, I know this. Yes!" I read through the possible answers and clicked one quickly. Always go with your gut feeling. Question number three was another I had seen before, either from the NCLEX 3500 or Nurse Lola's review course. I clicked right through. Question after question, answer after answer. Every single question that appeared on my screen, I had encountered some form or variation of it before. Yeah, the first one threw me for a loop, but from there on I was breezing my way through. I had the answers to them all. Dozens of the questions were word-for-word what I had studied. This was no exam for me, it was a review session. After about forty-five minutes, I approached question number seventy-five, the minimum number needed for the test to decide whether I was a capable nurse or an atrocity. I blew through the question and waited. Question number seventy-six showed on the screen. I started to feel anxious. How long would this test continue for? I'd known the answer to literally every question but one. Maybe I had bombed this test and was now in for a ride.

Question number seventy-six was feeling like something I had seen before… Yep, I had definitely answered it several times over on my practice exams. I chose an answer—presumably the correct one. The screen went back to the home page and informed me to contact the testing proctor. I raised my hand and waited patiently until the proctor came by and informed me that the exam was over. I looked up at the clock on the wall. I'd taken about fifty minutes to complete seventy-six NCLEX questions. The

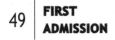

proctor walked me to the lockers, where I gathered my stuff and headed to the reception area.

One last ID check and I made my way out of the testing facility. It was still early in the day. I wasn't sure what to make of my experience, having coasted right on through and finished with near the minimum number of questions. I thought I knew it all, but there had been a time I thought I did well on a practice exam and totally bombed it. If there was any time for that to be the case, surely this couldn't be it. I wasn't in the right emotional state to be given the news that I had failed the NCLEX.

The NCLEX results are mailed to you six weeks after the test. These are the official results that most facilities ask for when you apply for a job. For a small fee, though, you can get your results online two days after your test. Though deemed "unofficial," they are accurate and generally accepted by potential employers.

Don't want to wait those two excruciating days? Well, back in 2011, there was a little trick I had learned about to check whether I passed or failed only a few hours after taking the NCLEX. From what I understand, the trick still works. Allow me to explain. After completing the NCLEX, you want to wait a couple of hours for the results of your test to be transmitted to the testing body. The computer knows right away whether you passed or failed, but the results have to be processed before the unofficial results are posted online and the official results are mailed to you. You log into the testing website (you know what I'm talking about, it's where you registered initially) and pretend like you are registering for the NCLEX, like you did the first time. You will have to submit your credit card information like you did before, and because there are no refunds, you have to proceed with extreme caution. You complete the registration and, in the process of loading the page where you select a test date, you may receive a variety of messages. The first message may be an error message stating, "Our records indicate you recently scheduled this exam. Another registration cannot be made at this time." This is a good message—it means you passed and you cannot schedule another NCLEX test. In this case, your credit card isn't charged again and you are not prompted to pick a future test date. This doesn't 100% mean you passed, but the probability is very, very high.

If the website processes your information and tries to charge your credit card, it may mean you failed the NCLEX. Alternatively, those who receive something called the "Candidate Performance Report" possibly failed as well.

If you are blocked from scheduling another testing date and you receive a message stating that your results are on hold, it means just that. At this time there's no guessing whether you passed or failed. This is probably the worst message to receive, because the uncertainty continues.

Again, this is just a little trick of the trade. It's been very consistent in determining whether I and others I know passed or failed, but keep in mind it's not official results.

I did this little trick the evening of my exam and received the favorable message. I felt pretty good with the odds heavily in my favor. By this moment, I still hadn't informed any friends or family that I had taken the NCLEX because I was still being cautious about failing. I just didn't want the extra stress. Once the two days had passed, I paid the extra money and got my unofficial results online. I passed the NCLEX. I passed after having to answer only seventy-six questions. My intuition was right—I knew all the questions that were presented to me except the first. The official results I got six weeks later told the same story.

CHAPTER 3

FAILING THE NCLEX

SO YOU FAILED THE NCLEX. THAT'S WHY
YOU flipped to this chapter, right? Or maybe you
just want to read some stories of people failing the
NCLEX. This book is a buffet; fill your plate with whatever
you're hungry for.

Failing the NCLEX isn't the end of the world. Honestly, the most difficult part of this process was completed when you graduated nursing school. If things didn't pan out the way you had planned, there's still plenty of hope. Generally speaking, you may retake the NCLEX a maximum of eight times per year; each retake must occur at least forty-five days apart; and you have to pass it within three years of completing nursing school. Not all states follow these guidelines, though—some have instituted their own limitations and restrictions for the NCLEX. Take Colorado, for example: You're allowed to take the NCLEX three times in three years, and if you fail through the third try, you have to repeat nursing school. Other states, like South Carolina, require proof of remediation after your first failure. Research your state's policy regarding NCLEX retakes.

In any case, if you find yourself on the failing end of the dreaded NCLEX, it's time to recoup and identify what exactly went wrong. Are you a bad test taker? Maybe you get anxious during exams and your mind goes blank. This is a common issue. Or maybe you know the content very well, but the framing of the questions throws you off. The best way to prepare, in my opinion at least, is to do practice questions. You learn how to answer the practice questions and you master the material they cover. There is a limited number of types of questions asked during the NCLEX because the content is focused on you being a safe-practicing new grad nurse.

Unfortunately, there are those who fail the NCLEX several times. Let me tell you a story about my friend Peyton. She was always known to have a few loose screws. She liked to party and really didn't take nursing school seriously. Throughout her time in the program, she had to repeat several classes. Luckily for her, she didn't go to my nursing school—they would've eaten her alive and she would've never been granted readmission. She liked to party, she showed up to class late, and just didn't treat the industry with the respect it deserved. She operated on her own time and no one could tell her what to do.

Surprisingly, she eventually finished nursing school. It was time to take the NCLEX. She scheduled it and didn't study at all. Instead, she partied in the weeks that followed graduation and showed up to her first attempt hung over. She failed. It goes without saying that her irresponsibility and recklessness led to that first failure.

But what were Peyton's excuses the second, third, fourth, and fifth times she failed? She had an inability to focus and was studying incorrectly. Her method of studying was to religiously review the material from nursing school. Passing the NCLEX requires an understanding of how to answer the questions, and memorizing class material isn't going to help. Sure, she knew the textbooks inside and out, but that was never going to save her when it came to the NCLEX.

Peyton continued taking the exam once every two to three months. She failed the Illinois NCLEX a total of nine times across a two-and-a-half year period. It was a combination of her lack of focus, her partying, and her refusal to study properly. Before having to go through nursing school all over again, Peyton decided to move to Minnesota and take the NCLEX there. She passed on her first try. What did she do differently this tenth time? She removed herself from the partying, distractions, and bad vibes. When she moved to Minnesota, she had no friends and nothing to do. She spent all her free time doing practice questions, which helped her develop an understanding on how to answer the questions. Peyton passed the NCLEX after answering around two hundred questions. That's still a lot of questions, but she passed.

If Peyton can be a nurse, so can you. I mean it as a good thing, I think.

Remember that the NCLEX is focused on the candidate being a safe-practicing nurse upon entering the workforce. The NCLEX is pass or fail. In their eyes, you are either safe or not. The truth is, there are those who answer the NCLEX questions correctly and pass with the minimal amount of questions required, while others have to answer all 265 and fail. Then there's the in-between, the gradient that exists between safe and unsafe nurse, and an imaginary line that divides the candidates. If you answer

220 questions and pass the NCLEX, how safe are you? Apparently, safe enough. When you work on the unit or in the field, you will know exactly what I am talking about when you meet a nurse and you ask yourself, "How did he/she pass the NCLEX?" As for Peyton, she's probably best fit for a nursing job behind the desk that requires her to memorize and crunch numbers. That would be safest for everyone involved.

CHAPTER 4

FINDING A JOB

MANY INSTITUTIONS WILL ACCEPT YOUR UNOFFICIAL RESULTS THAT you receive online two days after completing the NCLEX in lieu of an actual physical license when applying for a position. Keep in mind, though, you will still have to pay for your license and provide a copy to your employer when it becomes available. This is required usually within the first thirty to sixty days of employment, depending on the hiring facility and their policies.

Based on your clinical rotations in nursing school, you have a vague idea of what unit you'd like to start your career in. Different strokes for different folks. If you like pediatrics, go for it. If you like the intensive care unit, hey, why not? Don't let anyone tell you the ICU is no place for new grads. Any unit in the hospital is a respectable place for a new graduate nurse. You do want to keep in mind how the beginning of your career may shape its future path. Though not very likely, if an outpatient lab decides to hire you as a new grad, it may be difficult for you to migrate to a bedside unit position later down the road, because the hiring manager of the unit may see your skill set as the equivalent of a new grad, and hiring an actual new grad gives the manager an opportunity for lower-cost labor and the ability to train the new hire to the unit standards. Yeah, that was a mouthful, but hopefully you get my drift.

I strongly believe that the bedside experience is crucial to a new graduate's growth into a strong nurse, whichever direction the career may go. Whether it be cardiology, pediatrics, ICU, neurology, or ER, bedside nursing is imperative to the professional development of a nurse entering the workforce. Pick a unit or department that strikes your interest and apply to those available positions across the city. Be patient; don't immediately just take what you can get. You want to be happy in your position. You will thrive when you are on a unit and working the types of shifts that align with your personality.

Of course, it doesn't always work out so conveniently. In my case, I wanted to start on a cardiac unit, but there were no morning or afternoon shifts available. Whereas some hospitals still use the eight-hour shift model, the hospital I was applying at required twelve-hour shifts. And the only shift available for the position I was applying for was from 7 p.m. to 7 a.m. This was a problem. I am not a night person. I love to sleep at night and I love waking up early in the morning. That's when I feel fresh and alert. I decided to apply for the position anyway, to see what would happen. I had applied to several places across the city already, but a lot of those positions were looking for nurses with experience. This night shift cardiac unit position was open to new grads like me.

I got a call from the unit manager, who wanted to conduct a phone interview. We did our phone interview and it went well. I inquired whether there was an opportunity to transition to day shift in the future, and she said, "Of course, a lot of our nurses move around—just as long as you stay on the unit." I then got a call from the hospital's Human Resources department for another interview.

Don't take these interviews lightly. Dress well and keep all the extra stuff modest and to the point. Set the cologne or perfume intensity level at a minimum. Don't wear any more bling than you usually do. And most importantly, be well-groomed. It's okay to have a beard (male or female, whatever), just don't let it be full of crumbs and rats. After you get the job, you can let yourself go. (Note: I have become aware that appearance on the West Coast far more lenient than the Midwest and East Coast, again; I am just speaking from my own personal experience.)

I often see potential candidates showing up for interviews wearing faded jeans and smelling like Axe body spray circa 2003. This isn't an internship at a video game software company; it's a position that represents the values and ideas of a whole organization, and you may be the face of every complaint and compliment. Take this hiring process seriously, please.

Hiring managers are looking for those "meta" nurses who are overly aware of what they are getting themselves into and what is required of them as a new grad nurse. Yes, there are some buzzwords that may be thrown in your direction; facilities would like to see you initiate those words as topics of discussion during your interviews. Nursing is about collaboration—you learned this in nursing school. Talking about the importance of *collaboration*, *teamwork*, and the role those tandems play in the *efficiency* of patient care and *safe* practices will impress a hiring manager. Hiring managers will often have a list of words on a notepad to see how many you check off. In the year 2021 and beyond, the variety of the type of patients you encounter is incredibly diverse. You will meet Muslims, atheists, Satanists, probably a Pastafarian or two... the list goes on and on. Talking about the importance of *culturally competent care* will spark some light bulbs in the minds of the interviewers. Cultural competency has always been a cornerstone in nursing, and has become more relevant today than ever.

Let's circle back to my experience before we lose track. I completed the HR interview, where I did really well, and had one final interview with my soon-to-be manager. I treated both interviews the same. Now it was a matter of my hiring manager deciding whether I had the type of personality that would fit her night shift unit. All I can recommend during this final interview is to be yourself. Don't pretend to be someone you think they want you to be. If your personality doesn't fit the unit, it's in your best interest not to be offered the job. You'll have a terrible experience trying to gel with your colleagues, and the situation will create an unfavorable culture for everyone involved. You will fit in somewhere eventually, because you are the missing puzzle piece to a lot of units out there. You just need to be discovered. My manager hired me, because the night shift was full of people my age and she felt we'd all get along and be friends. More on that later.

There's a stigma attached to new grads applying to nursing homes and taking the first offer they receive. There are some things you have to take into consideration. Ultimately, a long-term care facility or nursing home can become a very complacent job. If you are a new grad nurse and you survive the facility beyond your first year, the probability of you working there forever is very high. The required skill sets of a nursing home nurse and an acute care nurse (working on a unit at a hospital) are very different. Navigating out of the nursing home system can be difficult for some nurses because floor nursing isn't too keen on hiring nursing home nurses. At the end of the day, if you are happy with being in the nursing home and not utilizing a wide variety of skills (compared to floor nursing), then go for it.

Some nurses graduate and pass the NCLEX and start looking for non-clinical nursing jobs. Good luck, because a lot of those jobs require clinical experience. You truly expand your skill set in the clinical setting, and having the clinical experience will better prepare you for some of those highly coveted non-clinical nursing jobs. Once you've gained the experience, you can go into

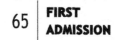

fields like public health, education, academics, research, quality care, and informatics. I know a lot of you will disagree with me, but I stand by my advice: Get clinical experience before transitioning your career into a non-clinical role.

Wherever you decide to work, make sure you place a lot of weight on the benefits that are offered. It baffles me when I meet nurses who, after everything they've gone through to pass nursing school and the NCLEX, still lack basic street-smarts. The most important benefit is healthcare. Make sure the facility you have interest in has a strong healthcare benefit. What kind of deductibles will you be paying? How often can you see a physician? Is your current healthcare team already in-network? Is the provided network adequate for your healthcare needs? These are questions that can have expensive answers if you don't do the research beforehand. You may find a nice gig that pays well, but what good is it if all that extra money goes right back into your healthcare because your needs aren't covered or the premiums (deductions from your paycheck) are unreasonably high?

Absolutely make sure that the place you want to work at has a 401(k) with company matching. I cannot stress this enough. You are only taxed on your income *after* 401(k) deductions. This is so important because it's an opportunity to begin building your retirement wealth. If your company matches your 401(k) contributions, even just a little bit, it adds up—especially when the market does well. You want to contribute at least 12% from your paycheck when you first start out and increase your contributions by 1% (or even 0.5% if they allow you to) every year. You can contribute a maximum of $19,500 (this number often changes, look it up) a year to your 401(k) to help lower your taxable income. 401(k) is a marathon, something you will contribute into for your whole working career. The market will go up and down, but after thirty-plus years, given the free money from company matching, you will retire with hundreds of thousands of dollars. If you find a gig with pension as well, then you are in the money. Don't ever give that job up. You'll be sitting on goldmine of 401(k) growth and pension when you retire. Some companies even offer stock options as well. I'll leave that to your discretion, because individual companies perform differently than the market as a whole.

Do you plan to continue your education? Your answer matters when deciding where to work. Some hospitals or facilities will pay for your continuing education or reimburse you a fixed amount yearly. When I graduated

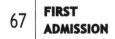

nursing school, I only had my associates in nursing (ADN degree). Obtaining my bachelor's degree in nursing (BSN) was important to me, and the hospital I was going to begin working for offered full reimbursement for your BSN. The only catch: You had to commit two years to the hospital. It was a no-brainer for me because I planned to stick around at least three years anyway. The same often applies to those looking to obtain their master's degree (MSN) or one of the varieties of certifications out there. You will save a lot of money by opting to work for a hospital that offers reimbursement.

Lastly, take into consideration the merit and reputation of the facility you are applying to. There are facilities out there that serve as a revolving door for nurses. The turnover is really high and nurses are leaving as fast as they're being hired. Do you want to be caught in that same funnel? Will working there look good on your resume? Alternatively, there are places where you'll encounter groups of nurses called "lifers." Lifers spend their whole nursing career at one facility and never plan to leave. They're happy and complacent, their work family is their life, and leaving for more pay is not in the cards. There's nothing wrong with being a lifer; in fact, a lot of them at a facility is a testament to how much nurses enjoy working there. In a perfect nursing world, you'd land a job with amazing benefits, awesome 401(k) matching, a pension, educational reimbursement, and yearly merit raises that are sustainable enough for you to stay forever. One could wish, right?

CHAPTER 5

NEW GRAD NURSING

SO YOU GOT THE JOB. CONGRATS! I'M **HOPING** you pursued and obtained the position you had your eye on. If not, well, enjoy your shitty, miserable life. Nothing is worse than waking up every day to a job you passionately loathe. You only have yourself to blame.

You got the position you wanted? Great, let's move on.

New grad nursing can honestly be its own source material. It could be its own book. With that being said, I'm just going to keep this as brief and to the point as possible. There's probably a fair bit of information I'll miss or skip over in this section, so don't come at me with your angry emails or DMs talking about, "Hey, I can't believe you didn't mention XYZ." Put whatever I miss on your shitty blog and people (not me) will read and comment about it. Thanks.

Nothing is more anxiety-inducing than that first day on the job. I'm not talking about company orientation, that was a breeze. Orientation teaches you all of the commonsense stuff you should already know—code of conduct, respect, ethics... you know, right? I'm talking about your first day on the unit, the day you worked so hard to get to. That first day on the unit encompasses all the hard work you put into nursing school, all the unfair clinical rotations, the mind-numbing politics, and your victory over the dreaded NCLEX.

What you learn rather quickly is that nursing school, your exit exam, and the NCLEX reflect less than 1% of the real nursing world. You learn how to be a "real nurse" in your first year as a new grad. When you walk onto that unit for the first time as a nurse in this highly coveted industry, you will realize that you have just been thrown to the wolves.

Luckily for you, you're not on your own. As a new grad, you will be paired with a preceptor (or a variety of preceptors) for the first three months or so. It all depends on your facility's policy, but most places train you for three months and then evaluate your confidence and ability to be on your own. We all know how you're going to show up on your first day: perfectly pressed scrubs, brand-new Littman stethoscope, your little notebook or binder for taking report, a pocket protector with safety scissors, a working penlight, and a sack lunch. Perhaps over-prepared.

You want to be prepared, but you always want to be relaxed. Let your preceptor lead the way. Your preceptor will serve as the foundation to your career. You are going to learn how to actually be a nurse, while also picking up all of your preceptor's shitty habits. Ideally, your unit manager picked a strong nurse to take you under her (or his) wing and to show you the way of the unit. Your manager wants you to be like your preceptor in many ways, but they also want you to be a young and fresh mind that will revitalize the unit. This is the truth.

Your first day can feel stressful, but in most cases, you'll just be observing the whole shift. Your preceptor wants to gauge your ability to learn and will probably spend this first day learning about you. First impressions are important, and if you are interested in learning and thriving, make it known. Ask questions, pay attention, and offer to help any way you can. Keep in mind, a lot of the veteran nurses are not interested in what you learned in nursing school. You're going to annoy them if you try to provide textbook corrections or say things like, "Oh, well in nursing school, I learned that so-and-so and such-and-such." You want to make friends, not enemies, especially on the unit. You'll learn why later.

As you navigate through your unit orientation, your responsibilities will grow with each shift. You'll begin to pass medications under the watchful eye of your preceptor and you'll enter clinical notes into the chart. The most mundane task, like making your first call to a doctor, will feel so intimidating at first, but as with most skills, you become better with practice.

Like most new grads, I was hired for night shift. The plan was for me to spend six weeks' orientation on nights, do two weeks' orientation on day shift, and then finish my final four weeks back on night shift. This would round out to a total of twelve weeks, or about three months—the typical orientation period.

I was paired with a tough Irish nurse from the South Side of Chicago. It was a perfect match, because I grew up around Irish Catholics on the South Side as well. We immediately understood each other's dry humor. She had been a nurse for quite some time and enjoyed being on night shift because it fit the needs of her personal life. Me, not so much, but I had to take what I could get. My manager did the two of us a great favor by putting us together. This isn't something that I initially considered, but personality conflicts with your preceptor can become a barrier to your learning experience or even halt your employment. Preceptors truly hold your fate in their hands. We were lucky that my manager saw a lot of common personality traits between me and my preceptor and knew that we'd be a great fit.

I walked onto the unit for the first time as a nightshift nurse on a warm September evening. I remember not having a jacket on that day and the sun being unusually bright for 6:40 p.m. It still felt like summer, which is quite a rarity by Chicago standards. I walked over to the break room which sat between the front desk and the back desk area and dropped off my snack for the shift—a protein shake, a bottle of water, a fiber bar, and a ziplock bag of almonds.

The unit was designed to hold about thirty patients, around twenty being the norm. Two patients per room, with the patient acuity divided amongst the staff.

I made my way back to the front and found my preceptor, Maggie. She was about twelve years older than me but in with the younger crowd. She smiled and looked at her clipboard. "You ready?" I shrugged my shoulders and said, "Yeah, I guess?" We were entering change of shift, so things were very hectic. Nurses from the day shift were trying to wrap things up and the oncoming nurses were looking for report. Naturally, call lights were buzzing and the unit secretary was trying to direct traffic.

This chaos is typical during shift change. You learn to adapt and handle it as best you can. Some nurses are flustered while others are calm. Maggie was the latter. We walked over to the assignment board to get a look at our patients for the night, and the nurses we had to hunt down for report. Maggie took one glance at the assignment and rolled her eyes. "Get ready to get shit on every night you come in." I would learn later that she wasn't speaking figuratively. Maggie hunted down the charge nurse for that day. The charge nurse is exactly who it sounds like—the nurse who is in charge for the shift, who hands out the admissions and assignments and acts as the mediator between staff and manager for the day. I heard Maggie from the other side of the unit saying, "You realize it is his first day on the unit, right?" The charge nurse made her way back to the front and double-checked the assignment. "He's smart, the assignment is fine. You guys will be fine. I'm off tomorrow, have a good night." The charge nurse finished giving her reports and headed out. "Ugh, she's a bitch," Maggie mumbled under her breath to me. Then she grinned. "Don't worry, we'll get her back. I'll teach you." Yup, my preceptor and I were a match made in heaven. I have the absolute utmost respect for anyone who looks out for me with such passion.

As a new grad on orientation, you and your preceptor will most likely have the toughest cases on the unit. This is mostly because you and your preceptor are viewed as two separate functioning nurses tackling the caseload a single nurse would otherwise take. This assumption is unfair, though, because the preceptor has to take more time for the usual tasks to observe, teach, and guide the new nurse. Having the preceptor and new grad take all of the unit's toughest patients can be taxing on the duo; but this will be the norm during your unit orientation period. All I can recommend is to tough it out and absorb as much information as you can. Even though most shifts will begin with an unfair, shitty assignment, you will even have some shifts that are blatantly obstructive to your growth. When you are given this type of assignment over and over again, you have to speak up and express your concern with the charge nurse—diplomatically, of course. If you allow yourself to continuously get dumped on, it will become a never-ending vicious cycle you can't escape. I have seen very passive nurses accept horrible assignments shift after shift and get burned out. They end up leaving, getting hired elsewhere for better pay to match their experience.

Maggie allowed a healthy balance. There were some nights we had awful assignments and we weathered the storm. My unit orientation period covered a few holidays, so we were fortunate to have some really easy nights. Don't ever take these types of nights for granted. These are the shifts that allow you to recharge your batteries and avoid burnout.

A lot of hospitals offer a new grad class, or something along those lines. It's a class once or twice a week for an hour or two where new grad nurses can discuss their growth and the obstacles they're facing. The class is optional (at least, at my hospital) and usually takes place before or after a shift in one of the conference rooms in the hospital. In theory, I love this structure. My experience, on the other hand, was not great.

The first class was informative and supportive. Led by the president of the nursing committee of the hospital, the class stressed to the new grad nurses that it was important to express any feelings of overwhelm and anxiety. I felt safe and supported. In fact, the number one rule of the class was, "Anything that is said here, stays here. We want this to be your safe haven." This enabled us new grad nurses to complain about assignments, preceptors, unit policies, and just things in general. But during the second class, I learned that the "rule" didn't hold water.

One of my classmates, a new grad nurse in the emergency room, complained about something very inane. It was a process with admissions and something along the lines of her not being fully supported and feeling alone in that process. Our class lead, the nursing committee president, who'd struck me as a very nice lady, grew very upset and said she would maybe bring it up to the emergency department. The new grad ER nurse immediately pleaded to leave the subject alone, that it was not a big deal. After a few minutes of everyone taking turns talking about their concerns, we took a break.

When break concluded, the class lead prepared to resume. It was at this moment the manager of the ER entered the room and asked to speak to the new grad class as whole. She stood in front of us, fuming with anger, and spouted, "Listen, I speak for a lot of managers in the building when I say that it is important to talk to your manager first about any concerns you have before you air them out to the world." She continued on, "You don't want to make a bunch of enemies as new grad nurse—" The class lead cut her off and asked to step out. We could all hear them bickering back and forth in the hallway. The president of the nursing committee sold out this new grad ER nurse, creating this uncomfortable position between her and her manager. The worst part, this happened literally minutes after she expressed her concern.

The camaraderie, the whole vibe of the new grad class being a safe haven, was bullshit. I was so glad I chose not to air any grievances about my unit, because I didn't want to be in the same position of this poor ER nurse. I never attended that class again. Weeks later, the president of the nursing committee ran into me in the hallway and asked about my absence from the class, and I informed her that I just didn't feel safe sharing my unpleasant experiences— and left it at that.

As the weeks pass and your responsibilities grow, you'll make life easier for your preceptor. You'll find yourself doing more while your preceptor scales back. This is often the tail-end of your orientation period, where you'll be building up your confidence to be officially on your own. Oftentimes, during the last week or two, you'll be on your own while your preceptor books vacations on their phone.

CHAPTER 6

HOLDING YOUR OWN

BEING ON YOUR OWN IS NOT AS FRIGHT-ENING as it sounds. The actual management of patients on the unit isn't as difficult as many make it seem. The real difficulty comes with managing your surroundings. During your orientation and precepting period, you and your preceptor probably received the first admission on the unit every shift. The excuse the charge nurse always gives is, "Oh, the new nurse needs to learn how to do admissions, get the experience, and become a master at it." It's partly true. Obviously, with experience and repetition, you grow and improve at a particular task. A great skill to have is to know how to navigate through your admissions.

Being able to take care of an admission in a timely manner can really lay down the foundation of the whole shift.

When you're on your own, it's a completely different story. Prepare for first admissions all the time. You'll walk into your shift, take a look at the assignments, and see yourself with the first admission. New grad nurses tend to be very passive, and veteran nurses or charge nurses can often take advantage of that. It's great to be helpful and willing, but it's not healthy to begin every shift with an admission. You never know what you're up against, and it can lead to a string of bad shifts and burnout.

The solution is as simple as speaking up for yourself. Accept your assignments when reasonable, and understand that not all shifts will be fair—the unit and patient load doesn't always balance out perfectly—but if you are routinely on the short end of the stick, speak up. Talk to the nurse in charge of that day's assignment. Oftentimes, the charge nurse is unaware of your string of unfair assignments because the charge nurse role is occupied by a different nurse each shift. It's not the charge nurse's job to figure out the landscape of past assignments, but rather, the individual nurse's responsibility to inform those in charge that assignments have been unfair.

I hate to break this information to you, but you'll also learn that your shitty assignments are sometimes deliberate. This is probably more common than the coincidence of getting a string of bad assignments. If you piss off a veteran nurse and later on, she is the charge nurse, you better believe she is going to get you back by giving you the worst four patients on the unit and the first admission. This is where "nurses eat their young." Veteran nurses want to see you succeed but enjoy the struggle and tears you shed along the way to success.

There was a veteran nurse on my unit named Elisa. She was barely five feet tall, but was able to see over everyone's bullshit. She was very proper, religious, smart, and Filipino. There's one like her on every unit. She was the epitome of old-school. "The devil finds work for idle hands" is a saying Elisa lives by, at least in reference to new grad nurses. She felt that veteran nurses should always have the easiest assignments and have earned the right to sit around all shift. If she caught a new grad nurse sitting around on their phone during downtime, she'd make a snarky comment under her breath. She felt every minute must be spent, and she despised any idea of efficient nursing. Efficient nursing didn't exist in Elisa's world; relaxing was only for the initiated.

Elisa was always torn about me. We didn't see quite eye to eye. She hated the fact that I was atheist and was annoyed any time I scoffed at her attempts to teach me about the Word of God. On the other hand, she was really appreciative that I had dated a string of Filipino women and that I was quite knowledgeable about her culture and customs.

Anyway, no one likes being the charge nurse because of all the headaches and politics attached to the role for that shift. For those reasons alone, the charge nurse role often gets dumped onto the new grad because a dummy new grad doesn't know any better and is too shy to speak up. Lucky me, I was that dummy one day. I showed up on the unit and found myself assigned as charge nurse for the night. At first, I was okay with it. The charge nurse often avoids getting any admissions, and it felt good to take a break from being slammed with admissions shift after shift.

Coincidentally, Elisa had switched to day shift for a couple weeks because of a personal matter. I'm sure you know what's next. Elisa was working the next morning, and I was in charge of the morning assignments. The idea is to balance out difficulty of patients amongst the staff coming on shift. It's easier said than done, because there are a lot of factors to consider: personality, skill level, who's returning for a second day in a row, and so on.

On this particular morning, we had four nurses coming onto the morning shift. Three of the nurses had worked the morning before and Elisa was joining them as nurse number four. Nurses almost always want back their patient from the shift before. It's easier to do charting and pass meds if you already know the patients and their schedules—it just makes for an easier shift all around to have all your patients back. Fair enough, right? Yeah, it was fair, to everyone but Elisa. That automatically left her with the first admission and a couple of tough cases. As I was putting the morning assignment together, I had a decision to make. Do I move patient assignments around to make it balanced for everyone, and piss off three nurses? Or do I just delegate a really bad assignment to one nurse, and deal with her wrath alone? For me, the answer was simple: it's better to have one nurse angry with you than to have three!

So I took a big shit on Elisa. I gave her an awful assignment and the first admission. I filled out the assignment board and waited until the morning shift came in. My plan was to give my report to the oncoming nurses and bounce the fuck out of there before I had to deal with how God was going to strike me down on my way home. I knew Elisa was going to be pissed, especially considering that her colleagues for that shift were all going to have it easy and she would have to watch them all relax and watch Netflix on their phones while she frantically ran from room to room for twelve hours. Yup, I suck.

My heart began to race around 6 a.m. I was just about finished passing all my medications to my patients and finished all of the charge nurse tasks. The ER wasn't calling for any admissions yet and everything seemed good to go. Six thirty rolled around and I felt like a nervous wreck. I was terrified of Elisa, and my fear perhaps was indicative of the mistake I was making. I knew Elisa was going to be pissed, but how long would it last?

The unit began to fill up with the morning rush. Doctors, secretaries, oncoming nurses, and patient family were all strolling in at 7:00 a.m. A few of the nurses came in, looked at the assignment board, and said, "Thanks Jaison, I was hoping to get all my people back." Elisa entered the unit with her coffee in her hand, a steel tumbler filled with whatever coffee she made at home. She was all smiles. Elisa made her way to the assignment board and noticed she was assigned the first admission. She looked over to me. "Charge nurse, what time is this admission coming?" Nonchalantly, I replied, "Oh you know, maybe around 7:30 or so, the usual." Elisa raised her eyebrows and curled her lips. "I see we forgot we have some younger nurses on today who can sharpen their admission skills." She then made her way to the break room to drop off her stuff.

I hastily gave my morning report to a couple of the on-coming nurses; luckily, none of my reports were to Elisa. I remember glancing across the unit and seeing Elisa receive report from some other nurses. The look on her face spoke a thousand words—she was growing increasingly annoyed at the level of difficulty of her assignment.

After I finished giving my reports, I went into the break room to grab my things. As I turned around to head out, I was confronted by Elisa. She was fuming. "You gave me a very bad assignment, Jaison. On top of that, I have an admission coming in a few minutes. Did you not learn anything during your orientation?" I tried to explain to her that the other three nurses had worked yesterday and it was easier to just give everyone their patients back. She didn't appreciate my answer and came back with, "Okay, that's fine, but you know God will get you, and if he doesn't, that means I will." Fucking great, now this woman is inflated with the power of the Crusades in the back of her mind.

I would be off for the next few days, but a colleague of mine texted me later telling me that Elisa had had one of the worst shifts of her life and everyone was so happy that I'd stood up to her. I explained back that it wasn't anything vindictive, and I simply played the poor hand I was dealt. Elisa thought I was after her, though, and I knew she was going to be after me.

Several days passed and I completely forgot about how I'd thrown her to the wolves. I walked on the unit, fresh and ready for the night shift ahead. Standing in the middle of the unit was Elisa, clipboard in her hand paired with a grin on her face. "Hello Jaison, you enjoy your few days off? Did you get all the rest that you needed?" I wasn't sure if her questions were rhetorical, so I shrugged my shoulders. "I don't know, I guess so." She continued on, "A superstar nurse like you is always ready for a shift like tonight, right?" I knew where this was going now. She continued, "I am the charge nurse today. The assignment is right here." I quickly glanced around. "Elisa, there's like two new grads here, and you hate being charge nurse. Why wasn't one of them in charge?" Elisa let out an arrogant, sarcastic laugh. "My dear, I volunteered to be charge today." I sarcastically laughed as I made my way to the break room. "Wonderful, fuck my life, right?"

I dropped my stuff off and took a deep breath. I was rested, but not ready for tonight's bullshit. I made my way out and looked at the assignment board and took down my notes. Elisa had given me patients all over the unit.

It's customary to keep nurses mostly contained to a certain area of the unit, so they can set up a station and kind of see all their patients' rooms from just one position. I wasn't getting that luxury. I would be walking all over the unit all night to keep an eye on my patients. I was already annoyed, but mentally prepared of the possibility of this being the least of my worries. I immediately peeked into all of my patients' rooms to get a glimpse of the night ahead of me. Seeing tons of pumps and devices is never a good sign. Strike two.

I jotted down the names of the nurses for my patients and hunted them all down for report. Elisa made sure I was receiving on-shift report from several nurses. Strike three. I found the first nurse, Claire. Claire was a busybody go-getter. Too perfect and Bible-thumping for our unit's culture, but you could always expect your patients to be in tip-top shape when you received them from her. Claire had on a fake smile as I approached her, which turned to a half-grin as she said, "You really peeved Elisa, she was talking about you all shift." I rolled my eyes. "Claire, just give me report so I can be done with tonight."

Claire proceeded to give me report for a patient that would need a blood transfusion in about two hours. She had done all the legwork; the unit was just waiting for the blood to arrive. Transfusions aren't difficult; it's just that they require constant monitoring and attention. Strike four.

I received another report (another messy patient) and then made my way to the last nurse, who was named Rose. Rose was a good friend of Elisa's, considering they were like complete opposites. Rose was gritty, liked to drink and smoke, and was as lazy as can be. Receiving patients from Rose was never fun because she often overlooked important information or would be really late with handing out medications, which would throw off the next shift's patient medication schedule. Regardless of her lackluster skills, she and Elisa were great friends and were barely related by some connection of extended relatives. Also, they were both Filipino, and that often matters—the older Filipinos like to stick together. Anyway, the last report I received was of an unruly patient who was hitting the call light all shift. Strike six, maybe? I lost count.

I earned myself a busy night. This was definitely the sort of shift that will burn you out for the rest of the week. In a matter of minutes, my well-rested-self unraveled into despair. It was only the first hour and emotionally, it felt like my night should already be over. Elisa was wrapping up her paperwork and walked over to me with a yellow Post-It note. "Oh, I almost forgot, here is your admission. The ER is very busy, so they'll be calling soon with report." Elisa had a big smile on her face. She had accomplished what she'd set her heart on and buried me. I was in for one of the worst shifts ever. I flipped the note around. "Substance-induced tachycardia. Observation. Alcohol." I was about to get a drunk who had snorted some cocaine and now his heart was beating too fast. This is the kind of patient who will be combative and unruly all night long. Great. Strike ten, if that even matters at this point.

I handled the night as best as I could. I ran from one end of the unit to the other trying to pass my medications and answer my call lights. My fellow nurses were very helpful that shift, but were also swamped with their own responsibilities. You'll quickly learn who your unit friends are. Those who are willing to help you when they're faced with similar problems are the ones you'll probably develop lifelong friendships with. There are others who will happily sit and relax all shift, watching you chaotically scatter back and forth on the verge of a nervous breakdown. Feel sorry for those nurses; they behave this way because they were once in your shoes and no one helped them. Killing your colleagues with kindness goes a long way. Being vindictive simply creates too many enemies.

My drugged-out alcoholic partier came to the unit a couple hours later. Luckily for me, this patient was held in the ER a little long due to some unstable factors. The delay allowed me to catch up a little bit, so when she appeared, I was ready for whatever was ahead. The patient was being rolled into the unit and, to my surprise, had a police escort. This was not mentioned in any of the notes or report. The officer came up to me and put his finger in my face. "You the nurse for our friend?" I sized the officer up and down. "Yeah, what's the problem?" The officer was just 100% done with his assignment. "Once this girl is stable, we're taking her in to the station."

I wheeled the new patient to her private room where she was handcuffed at the wrist to the bedside rail. I began my admission and assessment. It involves a health history and this and that—a bunch of questions the patient has probably answered a dozen times in the emergency room, but here we are, answering them again. I gathered some information from the officer as well. Due to the acute cardiac issue, she was sent to my unit, which was a telemetry unit—a unit that monitors patients' cardiac activity. This patient was a very attractive twenty-two-year old exotic dancer at a nearby gentleman's club. During her evening shift, she allegedly snorted some lines of cocaine, downed several shots of tequila, and stolen money from the club. She became belligerent and violent, and the police was called. Once the police were called, she jumped in her car and fled. The cops intercepted her a few miles away, where she crashed her car into a pole. She was a piece of work. She was still high on coke, too, and her drunkenness had deescalated from rage to flirtatiousness.

So, circling back to the cardiac monitoring. Many of you already know that on a telemetry unit, patients are on a constant heart monitor called telemetry. The telemetry is a five-wire attachment that is applied to five areas of the chest for heart electrical impulse monitoring. The telemetry allows us to identify any serious issues with the heart through the evaluation of rate and rhythm.

I was still a relatively new nurse and my comfort level with treating someone around my age and of the opposite gender wasn't quite where it needed to be. This kind of thing comes with experience and being desensitized to these types of patients. Remember now, I had to apply the telemetry device to this girl, which would require some navigating. This patient was unphased by my explanation of the telemetry application. I asked my female colleagues if they would simply apply the device for me so I could avoid the awkwardness. They all declined the request, not wanting to deal with a drugged-out drunk stripper, and because they had already helped me a lot throughout the night anyway. I was on my own for this one and that was okay, I need to learn how to handle these types. One female colleague offered to stand in the room to be a presence, though.

My colleague and I headed to the patient's room. The officer sat in a chair outside of the room, scrolling through his phone. The patient was still handcuffed to the bed. I entered the room and she smiled. "You gonna hang out with me all night, love?" I laughed. "No, no, I'm just here to get this monitor on you, and once we determine you're stable, you have a date with that cop out there." The patient looked at my colleague. "And what's her deal? You don't trust me?" My colleague rolled her eyes and crossed her arms over her chest. I got to work.

If you're skilled enough, you can apply the five leads really quickly and be in and out without it being an issue. This was my plan, as I didn't want things to be more awkward than they were. I proceeded to apply the first lead, and the patient immediately began to laugh, squirm, and joke around for no reason. My colleague shook her head in disgust, said, "Yup, I'm done. You're on your own with this one," and stood by the doorway. I pleaded with the patient to hold off on the jokes because the sooner I could get the device on, the sooner we could get her out of there. Looking back at the situation, it was probably in her best interest to stall. She wasn't going home, she was going to jail once she was determined stable.

I demonstrated the lead placement on myself and asked whether the patient felt confident in applying the device herself if I removed the handcuffs. She scoffed at my request. "Sweetie, I want you to put them on." I let out a big sigh. "I'm going to just demonstrate on myself and you figure it out." She found all this quite humorous.

After a handful of crude jokes from Miss Striptease, she had all the leads placed in the correct positions and the telemetry was beeping away. I checked the monitor and it was displaying some very suspicious activity, as if she was moving around a lot, but she was lying relaxed in bed. I asked to see the placement of the leads and wires. She lifted her gown to reveal very large, obnoxious-looking nipple piercings to both breasts. This had to have been throwing the monitor out of sync—they were probably magnetized.

I left the room and returned with a denture container and informed the patient that she needed to remove the piercings so they wouldn't interfere with the monitor. The patient asked that I remove the piercings for her. I raised my voice at her and told her that enough was enough, and this needed to be done now. I had the officer remove the handcuffs and the patient made her way to the bathroom while I observed from a distance. Piercings removed and placed into a denture cup, the patient was slow in her journey back to the bed. She was wobbly and I could tell that the drugs were wearing off. She then re-oriented herself and smiled. She turned to me and mumbled something. I leaned in, "What?" She then let out a burp, followed by projectile vomit—all over my neck and scrubs. Thank you, Elisa.

The reality is this: Everyone is bound to have terrible shifts and, every once in a while, wonderfully easy ones too. Unfortunately, you cannot please everyone when you're the charge nurse, and you can unknowingly put a nasty target on your back. Nurses will find the silliest ways to get you back. It can range from difficult assignments to efforts to sabotage your advancement. The culture is changing, though. Younger nurses are starting to realize that kindness goes a long way and is often the best way to combat a snarky, jaded nurse and the equally snarky, jaded work culture.

CHAPTER 7

PAY ATTENTION, OR DON'T; IT'S YOUR LICENSE

YOU'RE GOING TO SEE A LOT OF SHIT, and unsurprisingly, what you see represents only a tiny fraction of what goes on. You'll learn quickly that nurses don't like you in their business. They don't like you asking details about what they're doing during their shift. Nurses will tell you general things to keep you informed and at bay, but details are always left out. Nurses don't like to be judged by other nurses. Everyone has their level of work ethic, and it often doesn't line up perfectly with others'. There are many instances in which you just have to really pay attention to what is happening around you, because it can affect you.

I remember one time my unit hired a nurse with experience. She had maybe seven or eight years under her belt. Around that time, I was rounding out my first year. I was still on the night shift, with all of my work friends, and we were a nice tight-knit family. The new hire, named Melissa, was going to be trained by me and our veteran nurse, Maggie. Maggie trained me, if you recall, so both of us training Melissa would work out in her favor.

I had reservations about Melissa. She seemed a little off when I met her. Kind of dopey and unkempt. She looked like what you'd describe as trash. It was a little surprising she'd been a nurse for so long. Someone with her experience wouldn't be on orientation too long, maybe a few weeks. An experienced nurse at a new hospital really only needs to be trained on how to use the computer and the medication dispenser.

I had Melissa for a few nights, and she was beginning to prove me wrong. She was very independent and adamant about doing things on her own. It is what you'd expect from an experienced nurse, but because of her lackluster first impression, I didn't give her the benefit of the doubt.

A part of me remained cautious because she still rubbed me trashy and reckless. Whenever it was time to hand out medications, I insisted on doing it with her and observing because a lot of the documentation was still being completed under my account. I was accountable for any errors, since I was signing off on anything given to the patient. Still in my first year, I was rightfully paranoid. Melissa continued to insist on her independence.

After a few shifts with Melissa, she headed over to be Maggie's problem because I had a planned vacation to Paris and was going to be gone for the next ten days. Maggie liked autonomy, she appreciated the go-getters. So this new hire was the type of nurse she would like, except that she kind of felt the same way I did about her. Maggie told me that she thought something was a little off about this nurse. Anyway, she proceeded to train her for a handful of shifts while I was away.

While I was enjoying Paris, a unit friend of mine sent me a message and asked me what day and time I was landing back in Chicago—the unit manager wanted to know. I thought this was odd, but whatever, I gave her the scoop. A few days later, I landed home. About an hour after landing, I was sitting in a cab and my phone rang. It was my unit manager. "Hey, do you have a second to talk, it's kind of serious," she said with concern in her voice. I immediately got scared. "Yeah, what is going on?" She started to ask me details of my time with Melissa—"Did you visually see her pass medications, or did you let her go into patients' room on her own? How often were you next to her when she dispensed medications from the dispensary cart?" It was question after question about very intricate observations. I had just gotten off a seven-hour flight and I was tired... I thought maybe I should have a lawyer answering these questions for me. I just answered each question with the same reply: "I'm not sure, I don't know, why?"

My heart fell to the floor when my unit manager asked me to come in immediately or very early the next morning. I opted to go in straight away. If you're going to fire me over some bullshit, let's just do it now. I'll sleep better, I think. It was three in the afternoon and I rerouted my cab to swing by the hospital. As I sat for the longest thirty-minute drive of my life, I had time to replay every shift of the past month in my head. I tried to pinpoint the exact moment that I screwed up so bad that I had to be fired. I couldn't recall any serious patient event. There was no standout complaint that came to mind. I tried to think of maybe something I said or did to Melissa that would prompt her to possibly complain... Maybe it was the lack of autonomy? I also thought of all the hospitals I could apply at after being let go.

I arrived at my hospital and made my way up to my unit to meet with my manager in the conference room. My manager was very serious; she didn't ask me anything about my vacation. She asked I take a seat, then brought a folder and laid it out on the table. It was my medication report for my last three shifts which included Melissa's training. My manager had all of the pain medications highlighted. "Are you 100% positive you gave these medications?" I was jetlagged, tired, confused, and angry – but I knew for a fact that all my patients got all their medications. "Yeah, why?" She continued on, "Have you ever seen Melissa take any medications or anything?" I was pretty sure of this answer as well, because I didn't let Melissa really do anything except watch me. "Yeah, I basically did everything, she just watched me during my shifts." Then she asked for my opinion. "Do you think Melissa is the type that would fabricate giving medications?" I answered honestly, "Yeah, well, she looks like a junkie, so that doesn't help her case, but I don't know for sure." My manager continued on, "Okay, we are suspecting she has been stealing medications. She's pretending to give pain meds to patients and possibly pocketing them. A string of patients complained they never received their pain meds, when the computer says otherwise. It was none of your patients, though—we just needed to know if you knew or saw anything." Okay, so I was relieved I was in the clear, but pissed that I was there for this meeting that could've waited or been discussed over the phone. I thought about the situation for a moment. "So I'm guessing she screwed up Maggie's patients and documentation?" My manager nodded in agreement. "Yeah, it looks really bad. We might have to let them both go tomorrow." I grew angry at that, because I liked Maggie a lot and she had done a lot for the unit, including training some of the best nurses that hospital had ever seen. "Did you ever do any research on Melissa to see if she has a history? Maybe call her prior employers, references, or even Google her name?" My manager cringed. "No, that's where I slipped up. Maybe I'll Google her name and see what comes up."

I left the conference room relieved but angry. This junkie was about to take down a nurse that was giving her the freedom of autonomy and trusting her experience. I asked the front desk to call me a cab, since mine had left already. On my way home, I Googled Melissa's name. Her name was attached to several wrongful termination lawsuits. She had been fired from her past three employers and sued them all. I copied all the information and emailed my manager—hopefully this would help Maggie's case in the morning, but also, my manager was going to make a decision that was completely based on the events that happened on the unit. I didn't have Maggie's number, so I couldn't give her the heads-up, but considering how gossipy nurses can be, she probably knew all the details before I did.

I received a text early in the morning from an unknown number. It read, "Thanks friend." I responded, "Sure, who's this?" The number texted back, "Whatever you showed our manager saved my ass. I owe you one." It was Maggie; she didn't lose her job after all. Melissa's shady medication-passing only affected her own patients – and none of Maggie's. Maggie's history of being a stand-up nurse also strengthened her case to stay with us. I think she was reprimanded for not co-signing Melissa's medications that shift, but honestly, that was like the best-case scenario. When I think about the situation now, I don't think I had anything to do with saving Maggie's job.

Bottom line is this; don't trust anyone new. You never know where they came from or what their intentions may be. Learning how to read people is a skill you develop rather quickly in nursing because of the variety of personalities you meet. After you've worked several shifts with someone, and after they have gone out of their way to help you, you can begin to think about trusting them.

Reading people becomes an important skill. It goes hand in hand with your gut feeling, your instinct. My developed instinct would later prove useful. After a few years of working the floor on nights at the hospital, I took my talents to home care nursing. I mostly did it for the freedom and the money. With my agency, the average nurse was pulling in about $100k annually, and the hours were very flexible. For those that aren't familiar, home care nursing is a system in which recently discharged patients are returned to the community, and a nurse follows up with them in their home a few days a week. The purpose of the home visit is to complete a variety of tasks including wound care, obtaining labs, medication teaching, and post-surgical follow-up. When patients are home, they are mostly stable and it is very rare for urgent matters to arise. Some people love it (like myself), while others hate it. Home care nursing reduces the amount of rehospitalizations – which can save insurance companies a lot of money.

In any case, here I was, home care nurse extraordinaire. I was enjoying my life, driving around on my time and seeing my patients whenever I told them I'd be there.

One day like any other, I was assigned a new case and made a phone call to the patient. The patient's grandson answered. He was very cautious. He questioned the purpose of home care, inquired about privacy, and requested I park away from the house and enter through the back door to see his grandfather. He welcomed home care for the fact that it would replace the need for him to keep taking his grandfather to the doctor's office or the hospital (since the issue was manageable at home).

I grew cautious myself. I understand privacy, but the phone call with the patient's grandson left me with an uneasy feeling. He was too cautious, and for what? Their home was in a fairly nice neighborhood on the South Side of Chicago. It was a neighborhood that housed a lot of police officers and firefighters, though the patient was neither. He had lived there for over fifty years and was now elderly, around ninety.

I drove up to the house and did my usual precursory inspection to make sure all things looked in order. I checked the condition of the landscaping, windows, doors, and so on. The condition of a home gives you an idea of what you're getting yourself into. Per the grandson's request, I parked a few houses down and made my way up the walk. I could see the main living room windows were very dark, like they had tints on them; I couldn't see anything inside, even with the sun shining directly onto the home. I went up the driveway and into the backyard. The backyard wasn't the nicest, but nothing was of concern. It was obvious the yard and home hadn't been renovated in decades. I knocked on the flimsy screen door.

A few minutes passed before I finally hear footsteps making their way across the home. Someone leaned into the door and peeked through the window—presumably the grandson. The door opened to reveal a man in his thirties. He was balding, unkempt, and wearing a black shirt with jeans. "Are you here to see my grandfather?" I peeked around inside to ensure my safety, then said, "Yes, which way do I go?" To my left was the kitchen and the entryway to the rest of the home, and on my right were stairs leading down to the basement, which I had no business with. I entered the kitchen and the grandson directed me to a door next to the cabinet, which was in turn adjacent to the stove. "My grandfather is in there. If you need me, I will be in the living room. Just holler for me." The kitchen was such a mess, I was afraid to see what was next.

I headed into the room and saw an old frail man. He was sitting upright in his bed. Though he was hard of hearing, he was all smiles. He appeared happy and healthy for his age. I checked him out and provided wound care for some injuries he received from a fall. He spoke very highly of his grandson, who was standing in the doorway—I felt his presence behind me. Perhaps he wanted to assess the situation for himself. I wrapped up and headed out of the room to the grandson waiting for me. I discussed his grandfather's care and had him sign my paperwork, while nonchalantly trying to assess the rest of the home that was within my view. The living room was very dark and I could see garbage bags blocking the windows and what appeared to be stacks of computer servers in the corner of the room. The grandson made sure to be in my way so I couldn't fully see what was going on in there. Something was fishy.

I returned the next week for my usual care for Gramps. Overly cautious grandson led me to his grandfather's room and I began my care. As I made my way out I saw baldy standing in the doorway of the living room. I took two steps towards him for his signature and he immediately approached me. "Oh, we can talk here." He was clearly trying to directly my attention away from that side of the house. After some chit chat and an attempt on my part to sympathize with the grandson, he revealed to me that his parents had passed away in a car accident when he was younger and then he spent some time in California and returned home to Chicago to care for his grandfather, who was like a father to him. He mentioned he was lonely and had no time for a social life. Those are often the key ingredients to make someone who is up to no good.

Another week went by and I was back at the home to perform my visit. The grandson was comfortable enough with me to go about his business in the living room and not spy on me and his grandpa for this visit. I took care of my duties with the grandpa, but this time, I did things very quietly. I had a small plan in place. I wanted to wrap up as fast as I could and catch the grandson off guard in the living room. I needed to get a better look at whatever was going on in there.

I completed my care and quietly made my way out. Baldy was still in the living room. I walked in with my clipboard in hand, ready for signature. I wanted to play dumb and naïve. Baldy had his back towards me, he was facing several computers. The room was filled with black garbage bags hung and tucked around the sides of every corner where light could've gotten in, and there were makeshift tints hanging in front of the windows. There was a table standing upright at the front door—as if to block anyone from getting in. Photos of women everywhere. The photos were taped to the walls, on the floor; some sort of organization effort was going on. I looked down briefly and got a better look at the one of the photos. It appeared to be a young girl. In fact, all these photos appeared to be young girls. I couldn't guess an age, but they looked young enough to make me look away and feel uncomfortable.

Baldy leaped up from his computer chair and lunged at me. He grabbed the collar of my scrubs and forced me out of the room. "YOU ARE NOT SUPPOSED TO BE IN HERE!" I dropped all my things and was momentarily disheveled while he continued, "What did you see? You answer me truthfully." I felt my safety threatened, so I answered, "I don't know, nothing, I guess. I was just coming in to get a signature. I'm sorry." He signed my paperwork and showed me the back door. "You don't need to come back anymore; we'll manage just fine without you."

This guy may have been running some sort of pedophile photo sharing ring, or he was just a pervert and I was too much into his business. When I got home I searched his name in sex offender directories and arrest histories. His name and photo came up. He was a sex offender in California and had spent a year in jail for sharing photos of minors. He was back on his bullshit, this time in Chicago. I immediately made an anonymous tip to Adult Protective Services, 311, and the police precinct nearby. I also notified my manager of what went down. There really isn't anything you can do beyond that. A Google search a few weeks later confirmed an arrest for child pornography. Good riddance.

You can't help but feel bad for Gramps, though. He was nearing the end of his lengthy life and his grandson had been arrested again for his bullshit. I'm hoping he was properly placed in a nursing home and lived out the rest of his days playing checkers and watching old movies. Trust your gut. Follow your intuition.

CHAPTER 8

DEATH ON THE JOB

FOR A NURSE, SEEING DEATH IS INEVITA-
BLE. PEOPLE will often ask if you remember
your first patient who passed away. The first death
sticks with you through the immediate future, but as your
patient death toll piles up, you often forget that first one,
unless it was very memorable.

There will always be that one patient death that sticks
with you forever, though. More often than not, it's because
it was a patient you connected with or related to. When I
sat down and thought about my first patient death, I was
able to narrow it down to about two or three different patients. The memories of those deaths are somewhat foggy

and blended together, mainly because these patients were already on their way out and their deaths didn't come as surprises to me. But there is one death—not one of those firsts—which stands out in my mind to this day.

It was a stormy night shift and I was the assigned charge nurse for the shift. The emergency room was jampacked with complicated cases and they were overloading the intensive care unit, which was stationed right across the hall. We were about two hours into our shift and my unit was having a relatively quiet night thus far. The hospital supervisor entered our unit and called me over. We spoke of the current situation in the ER and the need for one more bed for a patient who would be admitted to the ICU. Since the ICU was full, they needed to send one of their patients over to us. Naturally, I asked that we get the easiest patient because we were not an intensive care unit and my nurses on staff this shift weren't equipped to handle such cases. The supervisor agreed and headed over to the ICU to figure out how we were going to play musical chairs with these patients.

I went over to our new grad on the unit and informed her she was getting the transfer from the ICU, and I'd consider it her admission for the shift and leave her alone for the rest of the night. She agreed to take whatever wildcard case that got thrown at us. The supervisor made her way back to our unit and gave us the patient details: a newly admitted twenty-five-year-old Hispanic male who had been in the ICU for just a few hours. It was believed he had severe pneumonia and had already started the treatment course, which included a series of antibiotics and the administration of oxygen via nasal cannula, or non-rebreather. Typically a pneumonia case would be sent to our unit before the ICU, but this patient's breathing was very shallow and his oxygen saturation was struggling to stay at a comfortable level. Thus, he was sent to the ICU until he could be thoroughly evaluated by the pulmonologist in the morning. The ICU chose to send this patient over because they felt his care the least difficult.

After about another hour, the patient made his way onto our unit. As the new grad got his room situated and comfortable, I decided to speak to the patient and fill him in on what was going on. I explained to him the situation with the emergency room and the ICU and elaborated on how he was best fit for our unit. He agreed. He was pleasant, talkative, but very much drained. He mentioned he was married with a small daughter and he was a dance instructor. He had no history of any illnesses and hadn't seen a doctor in almost ten years.

I liked this kid. He was very open-minded, intelligent, and understanding. There was no urgency or worry in his demeanor. The new grad got lucky; she got herself what appeared to be an easy patient for the night.

The rest of us on the unit got slammed. We were taking admission after admission into the night. At some point around 11 p.m., my new grad came to me and asked me to take a look at her ICU transfer. I went over to the room and saw that he was asleep and his skin was very pale, his lips slightly bluish. I immediately checked his oxygen saturation and it was at 62 percent. (Normal is typically anything above 88 percent, and below that is the danger zone; 62 percent is damaging to your vital organs.) I attempted to wake the patient, but he couldn't be roused. I told the new grad to call the rapid response team just to be safe. Considering the ER was slammed, the rapid response team wasn't going to be as rapid as they usually would be. In the meantime, I had the new grad raise the head of the bed and increased the oxygen to help maximize the amount he was receiving. He was slowly coming to, and I asked him to continue breathing through his nose and out of his mouth to promote pulmonary exchange.

I asked the new grad to continue monitoring the patient while I stepped away and informed the others on the unit that we had an active rapid response and the team should be up shortly. I suddenly heard my new grad shriek from the back of the unit, "CODE BLUE! CODE BLUE! CODE BLUE!" I dropped my stuff and ran to the unit phone and dialed a code blue while the other nurses grabbed the crash cart (a mobile storage device found on every unit that contains all of the necessities to run a code blue). As the code blue alert went over the intercom, the rapid team arrived with the hospital supervisor. A few nurses from the ICU ran over to our unit to help tend to our code blue. I ran back to the patient's room and my new grad was already performing CPR.

As the resident of the code blue team began to dictate orders, I noticed the new grad was struggling with her CPR; she was emotionally spent, and it was apparent through ineffective CPR delivery. I stepped in and took over for her and directed the hospital supervisor to be recorder of events. The ICU nurse that was previously caring for the patient was filling in the resident of the patient details. The focus at this moment was to simply get this kid stable again—all the other details could come later.

I was pumping away at the CPR, sweat dripping off my face. I kept a good strong rhythm while the code team intubated and inserted a central line into the patient. The minutes were flying by and we couldn't get him to start breathing again. The patient's parents arrived on the unit about fifteen minutes into the code. They were screaming and crying, asking what and how this happened. We didn't have any answers for them. I kept pumping the CPR. The supervisor began to cry while recording the events. I could see it in her eyes, she saw what could've been her own son's life slipping through our fingers. More medication was given and I kept pumping the CPR. I didn't want to give up.

The parents continued to cry in the hallway. The resident left the patient's room to speak to them while another resident took over the code. I knew this was it, we were letting the kid go. I leaned over to get a glimpse of the conversation in the hallway. I couldn't hear, but the body language of the resident and the parents painted the picture I needed to see. The resident told the parents that there was nothing more we could do. The mother fell to her knees while the father tried to hold her up, keeping himself strong. I saw my new grad across the way burst into tears—I could only imagine how she was feeling right now.

The resident returned to the room and took a survey. "Are we okay with calling it?" Everyone looked at each other in defeat. No one gave a clear answer, but it was apparent that this code was over. I kept pumping the CPR and through my exhausted breaths I muttered, "Five more minutes." Everyone turned to look at the lead resident; they seemed to be in agreement, but it was ultimately the resident's final call. I continued with the CPR; by now, I was drenched in sweat. The resident thought about it for a few seconds and slowly shook her head. "No." The ICU nurse slowly grabbed my arm and signaled me to stop. I looked up at the clock and called the time. "11:44 p.m." The resident stepped in and did a final pulse check and brief assessment, she looked up and agreed, "Death time, 11:44 p.m. Thank you guys for your hard work. We did everything we could."

The usual procedure of following a death was initiated. For us, it entailed the notification of social services, the clergy, and others. The family is allowed to spend a few hours in private with the deceased before we pack and clean the room. Unfortunately, our unit was full of patients, and we still had to meet their needs. This is where developing a thick skin comes into play. You are not insensitive for continuing the job you have to do; rolling with the punches is part of the job.

I pulled my new grad aside and explained to her that we could not lose focus and that the shift was only halfway over. I let her spend some time in the break room and she eventually came out feeling ready to go on. I felt bad for the new grad, because this seemed like a case that was going to be full of finger-pointing. Was this a patient the ICU should've sent over? Was this a patient appropriate for the new grad? What underlying issues were missed by the ER for this patient to crash and burn so quickly? Did the code team do enough? Did we do enough? This is nursing.

The rest of the shift was a very somber one and ended uneventfully. Luckily for me, I had the next few days off. I was deeply affected by this death for several reasons. Firstly, the kid was young and healthy and around my age; I almost felt as if I myself had passed away. I thought about all my loved ones and how it would have affected them. I guess it was just a reminder of how we take life for granted. Given the moment in time, we didn't know what the underlying issues were with this patient, so we had every inclination to believe he was someone that could've been saved. If he had stayed in the ICU, we thought, maybe he would've had a better chance at surviving. For weeks, I was haunted by the cry of the patient's mother as she was informed her son was dead.

I wasn't the only one affected by his death. The new grad thought about switching jobs. As a matter of fact, it was a big reason she would pursue becoming a nurse practitioner the next year. The supervisor talked about the patient for days, while others on the unit kept retelling the story like movie with a shocking ending. Days later, the hospital put together a panel discussion for the events that transpired because the gossip had engulfed the hospital. A lot of records needed to be set straight, and facts needed to be delivered.

The discussion was nice. It adhered to patient confidentiality while explaining (not in detail) that the autopsy revealed some issues with the patient that were beyond any nurse's control. The discussion allowed for people to share their opinions and established that the nurses and code team involved performed at a high standard. Though I was never able to confirm it, the strong rumor was that the patient had severe lung adenocarcinoma (lung cancer) that had gone undiagnosed, and his family had a strong history of cancers. This patient was going to die anyway—we just happened to be a part of it.

CHAPTER 9

THE ODDS AND ENDS

THERE'S AN INFINITE AMOUNT OF TOPICS THAT CAN be discussed in nursing, and I'm not here to provide you with an anthology of encyclopedias. This final section will discuss a broad range of topics that I felt do not require a chapter of their own or that I was simply too lazy to expand on. Let's not forget, this is a handbook. I wanted to keep it handy and efficient.

On the unit, there is a lot of stress and grief shared by everyone. Being a nurse is a passionate job, in a very passionate environment, and that passion often boils over into your love life. You may find yourself sexually attracted or interested in an otherwise "not-your-type." Nurses develop relationships with other nurses and doctors in the background, and it's all kept a secret because the older nurses and management frown upon this type of thing because conflicts of interest can occur and drama can spill out of the bedroom and onto the unit.

I recall working one quiet night shift with just two other nurses. The ER was empty and the hospital felt desolate. This was my favorite kind of shift. This was the type of shift where you can sneak into an empty room and sleep for an hour or two while your colleagues keep an eye on your patients. I was working with a colleague of mine who was separated from his wife. He was a young guy at the time, around my age—I want to say maybe 25 or so. He had married young and his marriage fell apart because life just happens.

I'd noticed over the past few weeks that he had become very friendly with one of the residents that would stop by our unit on nights. She was a really nice Vietnamese girl named Jacqueline and enjoyed hanging out and talking about Chicago because she was from Westminster, California. She had expressed a dislike of hanging out with the other residents because her class happened to be very arrogant and hard to relate to. I liked her; I thought she was really down to earth and I enjoyed having her hang out at 2 a.m. when the unit was at its quietest. My colleague, Keith, *really* liked her. He would always tease me with, "Hey, let me know when your friend is coming by." He projected his ambitions as my own, often saying things like, "She's cute, you should go after her" or "I bet you can't wait to see your friend tonight."

After weeks of innocent flirting, the two had begun to text each other explicitly. Around this time, my unit had an unusually slow night. I guess Jacqueline and Keith were waiting for a night like this. On my unit, we had room called the "nap room." It is exactly as its name suggests. It was a large closet with a soft chair and a few pillows and blankets. Sometimes, during the night shift, a nurse would sneak in and take a quick nap without anyone important ever knowing. I believe our unit manager was well aware of the nap room and just looked the other way. The nap room always existed while I was there, so I really don't know its origin. I'm assuming other hospitals have a nap room too?

Anyway, on this particular night, Jacqueline came by and started flirting with Keith, you can tell they had been texting each other moments before. They asked me to keep an eye on the unit and they proceeded to the nap room. They disappeared for about an hour and returned disheveled. I am not going to speculate or assume what may or may not have happened, but this continued on for several weeks until tension grew between the two.

The two of them were at odds. Keith was a little bit older and was in and out of his marriage, which had no clear direction, and Jacqueline was young and naïve, demanding the world from him. The two did a great job at keeping this relationship a secret, but Jacqueline took their stagnant status personally. When they shared a mutual patient, she would often direct Keith's calls to another resident or purposefully wait until after his shift to respond. They were like a married couple being extremely petty with their children caught in the middle.

One day, emotions boiled over. The Jacqueline came storming onto the unit and asked me, "Where is your friend?" In a situation like this, I am nobody's friend. I shrugged my shoulders at her and continued looking at my notebook. She made her way to the back of the unit to confront Keith. I wasn't going to miss this, so I followed her back there. She started pointing her finger in his face. "Are you leaving her or no? You didn't think I knew you were working tonight, did you? You think you can avoid me forever?"

I immediately stepped in and pulled her into an empty patient room. We were so lucky it was dark, quiet, and our other colleagues had stepped off the unit just moments before. This was an opportunity to keep this issue in-house, without extra people getting involved. I explained to her that she was being irrational and needed to be professional. Whatever issue they had needed to be addressed away from the hospital. I made her realize that this was detrimental to her career and could turn into an embarrassing situation that might be too difficult to recover from. She stormed off the unit. Keith thanked me and revealed to me that he was working it out with his wife, but was still caught in between both women. He was probably just trying to have his cake and eat it too – whatever, I don't judge.

Several days later, Keith and Jacqueline hashed out their issues and stopped their little affair. Jacqueline stopped visiting the unit, and Keith soon left for a better opportunity afterward. It was a good thing that their romance ended when it did. Sometimes emotions can get the best of you and it can lead to poor judgment when patients' care is involved.

As you work your way through different units at different hospitals, you'll notice a lot of secret romances amongst the staff. Many residents or older nurses like to take advantage of younger nurses, or you'll see some extra-marital affairs between nurses who share the same bedroom problems. The direction of romances runs through different departments and levels of superiority. My advice is to just avoid any work romance whatsoever. If you have genuine interest in someone, wait until they work on a completely different unit or at a different hospital. Even if the relationship proves to be stable and separate from work, the gossip amongst your colleagues may not be worth dealing with.

You'll probably notice or even experience first-hand; the phenomenon of nurses "eating their young," as I mentioned earlier. Older, experienced nurses often throw the new nurses to the wolves. They give new nurses the more difficult patients or those that require tasks for the experienced. This happens because older nurses went through the same type of hazing and feel it's appropriate to pass the torch. The hazing is disguised behind asinine statements like, "it's a learning opportunity" or "This is how you'll develop experience." Bullying, hazing, mistreatment, and emotional abuse is hidden in the idiom of "nurses eat their young" and is the culture that continues to pass from generation to generation. When you migrate into a position of leadership (as a preceptor or experienced nurse), don't choose to have a short memory like many nurses do. Remember where you came from, remind yourself of the difficulties you faced as a new grad nurse, and be the driving force behind the changing culture of how the industry views and treats new nurses.

Little gestures go a long way. My mom was a certified nurses' assistant (CNA) for nearly forty years. She was a nurse back in the homeland, but when she came to America, the conversion test was too difficult for her because English was her second language and she was unable to understand the questions. Only a portion of her education was transferrable, and thus, she was only able to be a CNA. Things may have changed now, but this is how it was in the 1970s.

One thing I vividly remember while growing up was my mom's generosity towards her colleagues and her unit. She would often stay up late to cook the unit some ethnic dishes, or she would leave for work early to pick up coffee and donuts in the morning. She didn't do this all the time, but she did it pretty often. Her staff treated her well and she really enjoyed working her hospital. It ended being the only place she ever worked. The camaraderie she had amongst her work family was irreplaceable, and my mom was never interested in seeking work elsewhere.

Things are different now. Nurses and CNAs come and go like the ever-changing breeze. They change jobs so much; it's not uncommon for nurses to know other nurses from different facilities. People will often say that "all nurses know each other." To an extent, the statement is kind of true—nurses definitely know of each other, because of gossip and such.

You can't avoid gossip, but you can avoid *bad* gossip. Whenever I worked through a difficult stretch, like the beginning of flu season (October and November), I would make time to bring coffee and donuts on random occasions to my unit, for both shifts. It didn't matter if we got along or if we didn't even know each other. The donuts were for everyone and I made sure people knew they were from me. Create good gossip about yourself, because you may not realize it, but nurses on other units or even from other hospitals will somehow hear about you, and it will only work to your advantage if you choose to seek other opportunities. And I hope you're not thinking, "Oh really? Donuts? That's what's going to elevate my career?" Donuts are simply an example of the bigger picture of behavior and generosity you should consider displaying.

Older nurses are very generous with each other. You will see lots of food being traded in the break room amongst that crowd. Take part—eat, enjoy, and most importantly, bring food of your own for everyone to enjoy. Ethnic food is usually a hit on the unit.

Generosity doesn't just begin and end with food. Strive to be the most helpful person on the unit, within your limits. People remember your generosity and will help you down the road when you find yourself applying for a new job. Someone will recommend you or recognize your name and more opportunities fall into your lap because of your small gestures.

Safety is something that is stressed religiously during nursing school and on the unit. It's arguably the most important aspect of this job. What a lot of nurses fail to realize is that our own safety needs to be considered as well. Too often, we focus solely on the safety of the patient and others. Your compassion for others can become the biggest danger to yourself.

As you may recall, I did a stint as a home care nurse. Patients in home care are sometimes high risk for readmission to the hospital because of their noncompliance with medical treatments and medications. When a nurse establishes relationships with patients in home care, it is imperative to be able to identify any potential emergency, for example if a patient does not answer the door. I was once seeing a very noncompliant patient who was a former police officer, lived alone, and had no family. It was just him and his dog. I was seeing him twice a week to educate him on insulin usage. He was a new diabetic and was still learning how to self-administer insulin correctly and safely.

After a handful of visits over the course of a couple of weeks, we developed a trusting relationship. The patient grew comfortable with me knocking on his front door and letting myself in, while he sat on the couch and waited for me. He appreciated not having to get up, grab his walker, and walk through his congested living room to let me in. In my mind, we had a clear understanding of this arrangement.

I remember arriving at the patient's home one day for our scheduled appointment. I walked up to the door and knocked and proceeded to turn the knob. The door was locked. I peeked into the windows but was unable to see anything. I walked into the backyard to look for sign of activity. I was unable to determine whether the patient was home or not. I documented the incident as a missed visit and sent a note to the patient's primary doctor. In the event of a single missed visit, we usually aren't required to react unless we see something suspicious through the windows or any obvious evidence of concern.

A few days later, I headed over to the patient's home for our next scheduled visit. I walked up to the front door and took a peek inside. I was able to see some movement, so it seemed that the patient was home today. I rang the doorbell and then knocked on the door and slowly opened it. I called the patient's name as I entered, the way I had done several times before and the way we had both agreed upon at the patient's request. I saw the patient sitting in his usual spot. He made eye contact and I greeted him with a smile. He immediately started shouting, "Who the fuck do you think you are coming into my house?" I held my spot in the doorway and reminded him who I was. For a moment there, I thought maybe his blood sugar was out of control and he couldn't quite remember who I was, but he reaffirmed he knew exactly who I was, and he wasn't having it. He continued, "You don't come into my house without me letting you in, you asshole!" I was disheartened. This went against our understanding, so I tried to politely make my case to him by reminding him of our agreement and my duty to ensure his safety. He then drew a gun from his lap. "I don't care what we agreed on, you don't come into my house without me letting you in!" My heart dropped to the floor. This man had lost his mind and I was going to die.

I immediately began to plead with him to not act in haste and started making my way backwards through the doorway. I didn't want to startle him. I want to make one thing clear—the gun was not pointed me. The patient pulled it out from his lap and placed it on his TV tray.

Still, the move was obviously suggestive that he was ready to use it on me. I feared for my life because I was unsure of the mental state of the patient and his behavior was unpredictable. I backed out the door and ran to my car, then called my manager to inform her of what had happened. My manager called the patient and spoke to him. According to her, the patient was completely coherent and he was requesting the police to file a report.

I still had a few more patient visits to complete, so I continued with my day after taking a breather at a nearby park. My intention was only to ensure my patient was safe and healthy, and I was only acting within our established boundaries. At the end of the day, you have to remind yourself that our own safety is equally important, and you have to operate in the best interest of everyone involved. I later found out that after the police were notified, the patient cleared it up with them; the police decided not to pursue any action because he had admitted I was acting within welcomed agreement, and he hadn't actually threatened me or pointed the gun at me. It was a wash. The police never requested to speak to me and there was nothing outstanding in my name.

What are your thoughts on this whole COVID situation? Assuming you're a nurse, you believe and trust the science—I hope. You'd be surprised how many nurses think vaccines cause autism and COVID is a scam. The handling of COVID situation in America has been an absolute disaster. At the time of writing this book in late 2020, we have over 500,000 dead, nearly twenty-nine million cases, and a president (who himself was infected with the virus) taking the whole situation lightly during his presidency. America is the laughingstock of the globe while our healthcare system is battered and its workers are suffering.

As a nurse, there was no right or wrong way to handle being on the front lines in 2020 and 2021. There was minimal protective equipment for many months, and lots of nurses were still contracting the virus, and later, quitting their jobs. I don't have the answer on how to properly navigate the pandemic landscape as nurse, but I will say this; do what is in the best interest of your health and safety, and that of those around you. I never considered myself a 100% frontline nurse because I work part-time home care and full-time insurance, so my personal thoughts on the matter aren't from genuine experience.

Don't take HIPAA lightly. We are fully into the social media age, and I see too many young nurses eager to dance and over-share their experiences in and around the unit. Going viral isn't worth losing your job. You will accidentally post something in the background that is a clear HIPAA violation, and there's no coming back from that. Equally, being nosey pays no favors. I have worked for organizations that treat and have access to the records of some of the most notable people in the world. If I were to access someone's file simply to fulfill my own curiosity, I would earn myself a one-way ticket to unemployment. Hospitals don't play around when it comes to patient confidentially and protecting sensitive information. A recent example would be the Jussie Smollett case. If you recall, Jussie Smollett was a not-so-well-known actor filming a television show in Chicago when he (allegedly) decided to stage a hate crime attack on himself. As the facts began to unravel and more and more evidence was pointing towards a hoax, lots of people took it upon themselves to try to play detective. A lot of those people were nurses and others who had access to Jussie Smollett's medical records for the evening of the attack. Jussie Smollett went to the emergency room the night of his alleged attack and had a full work-up completed. Over fifty nurses and medical personnel accessed Jussie's medical record to fulfill their own curiosity, and it cost them their jobs. There were no second chances for these people who were not directly involved in Jussie's case. It was a clear violation of HIPAA, and they paid the price. Use your head please.

CHAPTER 10

PUNCHING OUT

GREAT JOB! YOU'VE MADE IT (OR SKIPPED) TO the last section of this exhausting manual. I guess by now, you think I hate nursing. A love/hate relationship would best describe my feelings for nursing. The bad days will always outnumber to the good days, but one good day is often worth more than all the bad days combined. If your heart has no desire to help people, you will find your way out of the industry. Which then brings me to my final point.

Leave work at work. One nurse used to tell me, "Once you punch out, this job is out of sight and out of mind." It was one of the best bits of advice I had ever received, and I think it provides a fitting way to wrap up this handbook. Your mental health is everything. Whether you work twelve-hour or eight-hour shifts, no matter what unit you're at, this job is demanding. You often take the stress home with you. So, make time for yourself. Make time to decompress. Spend money on yourself. I know that part sounds easy, but a lot of humble nurses don't spend enough money on their own well-being. Get massages, do the little things that keep you happy—coffee or tea every day, collecting comics, seeing a movie, reading a book, whatever. Pick up a hobby and stick to it. Pay close attention to the older nurses around you—a lot of them have hobbies. Cocaine and alcohol doesn't count! I am talking about vacations, cooking, and things like that. Take your PTO. It's there for a reason.

Always leave work like you're never coming back. I don't mean being shitty and leaving undone tasks, or having an IDGAF attitude. I mean punch out, put on your sunglasses, turn the music up, and make plans for the evening. You deserve it. You've earned it. It'll make punching out for the final time that much easier. Cheers.

Oh yeah, and the cover of the book? That's future me; walking out of work the final time, with all admissions complete.

ABOUT THE AUTHOR

JAISON CHAHWALA IS A FORMER DINING AND HOSPITALITY writer and personality for various outlets in the Chicago market. After years of covering restaurant and food news, Jaison shifted his focus onto comic books, releasing the hit book, *Regards Ditko* in 2019.

Jaison has been a nurse for over ten years, with experience across platforms ranging from telemetry, ICU, ER, homecare and insurance. Unique experiences, both fortunate and unfortunate, were the inspiring factors for this book. Be sure to follow Jaison and all his happenings on social media.

<u>Instagram</u>
@FirstAdmission
@TasteWithJais
@JayMoney8518

Send all love, hate, products, and anything else you
can think of to:

First Admission
PO Box #1
Lemont, IL 60439

Media Requests/Speaking Engagements:
FirstAdmissionBook@Gmail.com

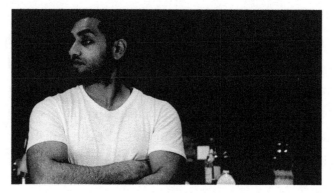

Photo by Brian Musial

Made in the USA
Monee, IL
14 June 2021

71252463R00090